PERSONALIZED MEDICINE

PROMISES AND PITFALLS

Gloria Gronowicz, PhD
University of Connecticut Health Center
Farmington, CT, USA

CRC CRC Press
Taylor & Francis Group
Boca Raton London New York

CRC Press is an imprint of the
Taylor & Francis Group, an **informa** business

CRC Press
Taylor & Francis Group
6000 Broken Sound Parkway NW, Suite 300
Boca Raton, FL 33487-2742

© 2016 by Taylor & Francis Group, LLC
CRC Press is an imprint of Taylor & Francis Group, an Informa business

No claim to original U.S. Government works

Printed on acid-free paper
Version Date: 20160301

International Standard Book Number-13: 978-1-4987-1491-4 (Hardback)

This book contains information obtained from authentic and highly regarded sources. While all reasonable efforts have been made to publish reliable data and information, neither the author[s] nor the publisher can accept any legal responsibility or liability for any errors or omissions that may be made. The publishers wish to make clear that any views or opinions expressed in this book by individual editors, authors or contributors are personal to them and do not necessarily reflect the views/opinions of the publishers. The information or guidance contained in this book is intended for use by medical, scientific or health-care professionals and is provided strictly as a supplement to the medical or other professional's own judgement, their knowledge of the patient's medical history, relevant manufacturer's instructions and the appropriate best practice guidelines. Because of the rapid advances in medical science, any information or advice on dosages, procedures or diagnoses should be independently verified. The reader is strongly urged to consult the relevant national drug formulary and the drug companies' and device or material manufacturers' printed instructions, and their websites, before administering or utilizing any of the drugs, devices or materials mentioned in this book. This book does not indicate whether a particular treatment is appropriate or suitable for a particular individual. Ultimately it is the sole responsibility of the medical professional to make his or her own professional judgements, so as to advise and treat patients appropriately. The authors and publishers have also attempted to trace the copyright holders of all material reproduced in this publication and apologize to copyright holders if permission to publish in this form has not been obtained. If any copyright material has not been acknowledged please write and let us know so we may rectify in any future reprint.

Visit the Taylor & Francis Web site at
http://www.taylorandfrancis.com

and the CRC Press Web site at
http://www.crcpress.com

Contents

Author

Dr. Gloria Gronowicz earned her PhD in biology from Columbia University, New York, and later obtained a postdoctoral fellowship in the Department of Biochemistry at the University of Chicago. She came to the University of Connecticut Health in 1983 as a postdoctoral fellow and later joined the Department of Orthopedics, where she became director of Orthopedic Research from 1989 to 2007 and developed the basic research curriculum course for orthopedic residents. She was a tenured professor in 2002. Later, she joined the Department of Surgery in 2007 and continued as a full professor with a joint appointment in orthopedics until 2015 when she became professor emeritus. Dr. Gronowicz has published over 100 articles in peer-reviewed journals, and nine book chapters. She was the director of the Center for Bone Histology and Histomorphometry, which she developed in 1998. The Center closed in 2007 when she joined the Department of Surgery. She has trained over 25 PhD and postdoctoral fellows, and is a member of the Skeletal Biology and Regeneration graduate program of which she was director from 2012 to 2014. Dr. Gronowicz also had major teaching commitments in the Medical and Dental Schools throughout her academic career. She received continuous NIH (National Institutes of Health) funding for the past 25 years and also been funded by numerous scientific and medical foundations. Dr. Gronowicz has served on NIH and NASA (National Aeronautics and Space Administration) study sections, and has lectured all over the world. She played major roles in the American Society of Bone and Mineral Research, and in the Orthopaedic Research Society where she was elected chairman of the Bone Topic Committee from 2012 to 2014. Her research encompasses bone biology, aging, response of bone to implant materials, otosclerosis, and integrative medicine.

Cover artist

Janine Gelineau is an award-winning professional photographer with 30+ years of experience in both photography and design. She lives in Connecticut and enjoys designing and creating book covers. She can be reached at a1bookcover@gmail.com.

Introduction

Radiant red, yellow, green, blue, and violet across the sky startle me as I exit my car and look up. As I lock my car, I think I see the rainbow reflected in the window again, but no, it is coming from another section of the sky. With amazement I realize there are two rainbows in two separate parts of the sky. This must be a good omen on such a terrible day in my life. Forty-five minutes ago, my doctor called me at home to tell me that my biopsy came back positive for breast cancer. He already made an appointment with me for tomorrow at 12:00, and surgery is scheduled for next week. In the end, the diagnosis was stage 2 breast cancer, estrogen receptor positive, progesterone receptor positive, HER2 negative. All of the biological features of my cancer and some of my treatments for the disease are part of personalized medicine. Personalized medicine is what I have accepted as my task to explain in this book, hopefully to help others make informed decisions about themselves and their loved ones. I also hope to transfer some of my great love and enthusiasm for human biology.

In general, personalized medicine seeks to identify the genetic, phenotypic, or environmental factors that influence a person's health risks. The genetics of my family told me that there was no family history of breast cancer of which I was aware. Phenotypically (observable characteristics), I am different in that I have a birthmark—vascular/capillary nevus or strawberry mark—on my face and legs. My nevus is an excess of blood vessels in the skin, and it can predispose me to make hemangiomas—benign tumors—of blood vessels filled with blood. Would this influence my chance of getting breast cancer? This is not known since the nevus is considered benign and not inherited. In addition, due to internal bleeding probably from one of these hemangiomas in my intestine, I have taken large doses of iron all my life to offset my anemia. There is now evidence that too much iron can predispose a person to cancer, which we will talk about in Chapter 4. My environmental risk is that I live in one of the states with the greatest percentages of breast cancer in the United States, and in a town with the greatest risk in my state. We do not know the cause of breast cancer or why my state has one of the highest rates of breast cancer. The other environmental issue is that my job and life are stressful. Stress is a great promoter of disease, since it affects our immune system and makes us more susceptible to disease. The other goal of personalized medicine is to create or find the most appropriate type and dose of medication and/or intervention to deal with a person's health issue. What happened in my medical treatment for breast cancer will be discussed later in this book.

As a professor in the Department of Surgery at the University of Connecticut Health Center, my work encompasses research and teaching. I earned a PhD in cell and molecular biology from Columbia University in New York City. When I came to the University of Connecticut Health Center, I started as a postdoctoral fellow and worked my way up the ladder to full professor. I like to discover new solutions to biological issues, which has been what I have done in my research and in teaching medical, dental, and graduate students, and residents at the University of Connecticut Health Center. As a biologist, the topics in personalized medicine also reinforce my amazement in human biology, in addition to animal biology, which shares many features with human biology. The structure and function of our bodies become even more amazing in their ability to coordinate all of the biological factors associated with these topics, and it also seems easier to understand why such complicated systems as our bodies can differ so much from each other. It explains how things can go wrong, especially as we age, and also how diseases can develop.

Personalized medicine is an emerging idea in modern medicine in the United States and appears to be driven by pharmaceutical and medical device companies. The U.S. Food and Drug Administration (FDA) defined personalized medicine as providing "the right patient with the right drug at the right dose at the right time. More broadly, 'personalized medicine' may be thought of as the tailoring of medical treatment to the individual characteristics, needs, and preferences of a patient during all stages of care, including prevention, diagnosis, treatment, and follow-up. Consistent with FDA's core mission, the agency is working in collaboration with researchers, manufacturers of drugs, medical devices and biologics, healthcare professionals, and others to better understand and adapt to the promise of personalized medicine."*

Interestingly, this definition of personalized medicine emphasizes collaboration with drug and medical device manufacturers, rather than accentuating the patient–doctor relationship for disease treatment and well-being in personalized medicine.

The administration at my institution has stressed the development of new techniques and pharmaceuticals—along with the study of genomics in research laboratories—as important for enacting personalized medicine at the University of Connecticut Health Center. If you speak to patients and the public-at-large, people define personalized medicine as more attention and time with their doctor, who would tailor their medical treatment to their needs and deal with all aspects of their personal health. In fact, hospitals and many private physicians have decreased the time they spend with their patients from 10 or even 5 years ago, so that they can see more patients and be able to receive reimbursement for the treatment of those patients, which has been the demand of

---

* http://www.fda.gov/ScienceResearch/SpecialTopics/PersonalizedMedicine/ucm20041021.htm.

the administration, insurance companies, and the government. Can that gap between patients' and doctors' perceptions of personalized medicine be resolved?

Another issue in personalized medicine is that medical specialties have become more focused on only one aspect of a person's health (for example, the gastrointestinal [GI] tract or bone health), rather than a holistic approach of the whole person and all aspects of their mind and body. The complexity of the GI tract or the skeleton requires doctors to specialize in these areas as separate disciplines of GI or orthopedics to be able to apply all of the knowledge of that one organ or system and its therapeutics for solving a patient's medical problem. A physician cannot be an expert in all aspects of medicine. However, our health is a combination of many organs and factors in our body, thus a holistic approach to health is critical for providing a better view of any disease that affects multiple organs. A holistic approach in medicine also provides multiple and multifaceted approaches to improving a person's health. The patient–doctor relationship is critical for the patient to heal. Therefore, communication among medical disciplines is essential if this personalized medicine model is to be successful.

By explaining the many topics in personalized medicine and the science behind them, perhaps we can come to an understanding of personalized medicine and our role in our own health. Patients need to take ownership of their health through better life choices in order to heal themselves. Specific aspects of personalized medicine may be important to pursue for the future of medicine, because this work increases our knowledge of disease processes that may lead to a breakthrough in the development of a new therapy many years from now. However, the more we explore human biology in personalized medicine, the more we understand how difficult it is to predict with certainty a patient's likelihood of developing a disease or the future quality of their health. The patient's role in his or her own health becomes more important since medicine and science will not have all of the answers to improve health, and the active involvement of the patient in healthy life choices is very important. Besides personalized medicine, is there another approach(s) to our medical system that would improve the health of individuals? To try to answer this question, we will start with assessing the state of our medical system.

In 2000, the World Health Organization (WHO) ranked the U.S. medical care system 37th in terms of health (disability-adjusted life expectancy), responsiveness (speed of service, protection of privacy, and quality of amenities), and fair financial contribution. Due to the controversy of these rankings, WHO did not rank medical care systems in the world in their report in 2010. In 2014, Bloomberg.com rated the U.S. as 47th in the world, largely because the United States has the second most expensive healthcare cost per capita in the world, but it is also starting to fail in the other categories. Will personalized medicine help the quality and expense of our medical care system compared to the rest of the world? The purpose of this book is to show the promise of personalized medicine in developing new knowledge and medical technology, but also to show the pitfalls in this new approach.

In the end, we must decide whether this new goal of personalized medicine can improve our health and lives. Will personalized medicine be cost effective and more responsive to patients' needs, improve the timeliness of our treatments, and be able to preserve our individual privacy? As consumers and patients, we must be the ones to make informed decisions on what is best for our health and our country. We cannot leave these decisions to the pharmaceutical and medical device companies, or even to the scientific and medical community, because of the conflict of interest to maintain their own jobs. Too much greed and desire for wealth at others' expense have permeated our businesses and society. Yet we want to see that our doctors have the best tools to help us survive.

Personalized medicine draws its foundation from a variety of fields, such as genomics, proteomics, epigenetics, stem cells, and biostatistics/bioinformation. These scientific terms form another language that can be complicated at times, since new terms and techniques are constantly being developed in science. However, once we understand the language and can "read" about it, we can better understand what personalized medicine offers us. A comprehensive glossary has been included in this book so we can understand this new language. Personalized medicine also includes integrative medical techniques, such as nutrition, acupuncture, yoga, etc. To find a specific therapy for a particular patient, extensive testing for the disease and the biostatistics/bioinformational methods to evaluate these tests are required. The costs for these new tests must also be considered in order to determine their efficacy in diagnosing disease with the fewest false results and in assessing the health status of individual patients. What changes to our medical system must occur in order to provide the best treatment for individuals? Is personalized medicine what we should be striving for? How should we improve the quality, expense, and timeliness of our medical care? What is most important? This book was written to start this discussion and find more effective approaches to improving medical care for all.

Ethics is also a very important topic in personalized medicine. Ethics is needed in order to guard the privacy of our personal medical information. If we are to sequence everyone's genes, then how should we protect this information and who should know about it? There is also the ethical dilemma of certain medical practices that may be difficult to accept by all people with different beliefs. Ethics and the respect for a patient's privacy and beliefs are required for medical doctors and personnel when dealing with a person's medical issues. How do we train new doctors in personalized medicine to learn all of these new approaches and be comprehensive in presenting to patients all of the different treatment options, including some therapies that show promise but are not mainstream and yet may be effective for them? How can our medical workforce maintain the highest code of ethics and navigate our medical system with its monetary emphasis?

Genomics, proteomics, metabolomics, epigenetics, stem cells, integrative medical procedures, biostatistics/bioinformational methods, and ethics will be discussed in separate chapters. However, a brief history and discussion of each chapter's topic will be introduced here, starting with DNA, the backbone of life. The discovery of the structure of DNA in 1953 revolutionized the scientific world and resulted in the 1962 Nobel Prize for physiology or medicine being jointly awarded to James Watson, Francis Crick, and Maurice Wilkins. Wilkins's colleague, Rosalind Franklin, who died of ovarian cancer at the age of 37, could not be honored because the Nobel Prize can be awarded only to the living and only to three investigators. Franklin used x-ray diffraction to determine the structure of DNA, independent of Watson and Crick, but they used the knowledge gained from her work without her permission to determine the exact double helix structure of DNA (Fuller 2003). This discovery was followed by the 1958 Nobel Prize in chemistry being awarded to Fred Sanger for determining the structure of proteins, specifically the protein insulin, being composed of particular amino acids. Since all proteins have an amino acid sequence determined by the DNA in our genes, the discoveries of DNA and the amino acid sequences of proteins are fundamental to our understanding of human physiology. Chapter 1 discusses DNA, genes, and their expression, which are crucial for understanding an individual's physiology and health risks.

The study of single genes is the primary focus of the field of molecular biology in genetics. Genomics, which is a part of genetics, is important in the development of personalized medicine, and this term describes DNA sequencing and mapping. A new interdisciplinary field, bioinformatics, has been developed for storing, retrieving, organizing, and analyzing the large amount of data generated by genomic applications to humans. With bioinformatics, we can analyze the structure and function of all of the genes (the genome) in an organism such as ourselves and use it in medicine. Genomics also includes the study of events that modify the DNA and its expression. The field of genomics has profound consequences to all of science. At this point in time, the U.S. medical care system is in serious trouble. Personalizing medical treatments and sequencing individual genomes may not be the answer to our problems due to the complexity of many of our chronic diseases, such as diabetes, osteoporosis, and heart disease (discussed in Chapters 2 and 3) and due to the complex biological processes involved in these diseases.

As a personalized example of the impact of genomics, this new era of genomics has had a significant impact on my own research program at the University of Connecticut Health Center. My university has partnered with The Jackson Laboratory for Genomic Medicine to build a research facility on our campus. The State of Connecticut contributed approximately $291 million in construction loans and research partnerships, and $809 million came from the federal government in research grants to The Jackson Laboratory (http://biosciencect.uchc.edu/jackson_laboratory). The hope is that this partnership will bring jobs and revenue to our state and university. The Jackson Laboratory is an independent biomedical research institution with its headquarters in Maine. It wants to lead the development of new medical treatments for personalized medicine based on each patient's unique genetics. All of the emphasis in research and new faculty positions will be geared to The Jackson Laboratory, superseding almost everything else we are doing, since we are a small research facility and hospital. This change is exciting, but means that most of us at the University of Connecticut will have to change our research emphasis in order to collaborate with Jackson Laboratory, because many of the resources available at my institution will be prioritized for this collaboration. Interestingly, according to Wikipedia, the word "genome" (from the German *Genom*, attributed to Hans Winkler) was in use in English as early as 1926. The term "genomics" was coined by Dr. Tom Roderick, a geneticist at The Jackson Laboratory (Bar Harbor, Maine), over beer at a meeting held in Maryland on the mapping of the human genome in 1986 (Yadav 2007). One of the starting points for genomics was The Jackson Laboratory. My university partnering with The Jackson Laboratory has become a major testing ground for this new genomics approach to medicine. Other universities and medical institutions nationwide are also embracing the genomics approach to disease and medical treatment.

Influenced by the term "genomics," scientists in protein chemistry coined the term "proteomics," which is the study of proteins and their structure, function, and activities. There are estimated to be 20,000–25,000 human protein-coding genes in the human genome. Often, proteomics, just like genomics, refers to the large-scale analysis of proteins, and not just one protein. Along with the analysis of proteins made in the human body, knowledge of their function, and which biomarkers or metabolites can be used to identify specific biological processes— both healthy and unhealthy—are needed. Metabolites are small molecules that participate in chemical processes occurring in the body, and they are necessary for the maintenance, growth, and normal function of cells and tissues. From this term has come the term "metabolomics," which is the scientific field that studies the chemical processes involving metabolites. For example, an excess of the metabolite sugar/glucose in your urine would demonstrate that you may have diabetes. Further analysis of the metabolites and factors in the blood can give a doctor more information on a patient's diabetic status and so help regulate diabetes.

Proteomics also refers to the interdependency of genes/genomics with proteins, and it became even more important with the completion of the Human Genome Project. The Human Genome Project was an international scientific research project aimed at determining the sequence and mapping of base pairs that make up human DNA. The project started with the U.S. Department of Energy's Office of Health and Environmental Research and became the world's largest collaborative biological project (Tripp and Grueber 2011). International government-sponsored sequencing was performed in research universities and centers around the world, including China, the United Kingdom, France, Germany, Japan, and Spain (http://www.genome.gov/11006943). It was a $3.8 billion investment that led to a $796 billion impact on our economy and the creation of 30,000 jobs. It is the world's largest collaborative project in biology. Charles DeLisi, David Galas, Aristides Patrinos, and James Watson of Nobel Prize fame were some of the people who were influential in directing this project. Francis Collins succeeded Watson and assumed the role of Project Head as Director of the U.S. National Institutes of Health (NIH) National Human Genome Research Institute. A working draft of the genome was announced in 2000 and was completed in 2003, but further analysis and changes are still being published. Knowing the DNA sequence does not always tell us which proteins will be formed. Thus, protein-coding genes and their functions still need to be elucidated in order to determine which diseases are caused by specific problems in gene expression and how to develop a therapy for the problem.

In addition to the DNA sequence, which determines a gene and its inheritance from one generation to another, gene activity can be modified by other inherited processes not involving DNA. This further complicates our ability to analyze someone's genes and be able to predict the likelihood for a particular disease. Epigenetics is the part of genetics that describes the processes that cause heritable changes and/or stable long-term alterations in gene activity that are not due to changes in DNA sequence. A more thorough description of epigenetics is given in Chapter 3. An example of the importance of epigenetics comes in energy metabolism. The fat mass and obesity-associated (FTO) gene affects human obesity and energy levels, thus affecting many processes in our body. Scientists discovered that the FTO gene codes for a protein that is able to change the expression of a multitude of different RNAs through demethylation, a process that alters many RNAs involved in protein synthesis (Jia et al. 2011; Wang et al. 2014) (see Chapter 3 for a discussion of epigenetics). Thus, the activity of our genes is modified by processes that are not directly related to the DNA sequence, but are inherited traits.

Another controversial topic influencing the medical/scientific professions is stem cells. Stem cells are unspecialized cells in the body that have the ability to renew themselves and even stay dormant until they are needed to regenerate a tissue on a limited basis. When required, they have the ability to develop into almost any kind of cell with special functions. Some stem cells, such as in the gut, help to repair and replenish the different types of cells in the gut. Other tissues, such as the heart, use stem cells only when there is injury to them. Of course, when the damage is too great, stem cells cannot successfully repair everything.

There are two types of stem cells: embryonic stem cells and non-embryonic "adult" or "somatic" stem cells. Embryonic stem cells are very exciting since they can be used to repair injured or diseased tissues. Adult stem cells have a more limited capacity to repair tissue. Controversy has developed from the origin of embryonic stem cells, which are derived from human embryos created in the laboratory from in vitro fertilization procedures. The use of human embryos for science is against some religious and/or moral viewpoints. To deal with this controversy, a new type of stem cell has been developed, called induced pluripotent stem cells (iPSCs), which will be discussed in Chapter 7. Much more scientific work needs to be performed in order to completely understand stem cells and to apply cell-based therapies to diseased and injured tissues, which is also referred to as regenerative or reparative medicine.

If we are to have personalized medicine, then we must include integrative medicine, such as nutrition, acupuncture, yoga, energy medicine, and meditation, to name a few of the techniques that complement our more pharmaceutical- and device-oriented approaches to medicine. These more "natural" treatments are also important for our health and well-being, and are able to alleviate stress and combat disease. These topics, along with other integrative medical techniques, will be discussed at length in Chapters 4 and 5.

Many of these integrative medical approaches are thought to prevent or delay the onset of disease. How valuable are these integrative medicine approaches to our health and well-being? I hope to convince you that they are essential so that we can create a more cost-effective program for our own health and contribute to driving down the costs of our medical system. However, many of these therapies require our active participation outside of the doctor's office to help us heal or stay well. Some of these integrative medical treatments or programs also require our own financial investment, since they are not reimbursed by our medical system. Should we create a medical system with more emphasis on preventative medicine and reimbursement for the evidence-based integrative techniques that are effective? It appears that there are a great number of people in medicine and science who believe that this is an important road to take, especially with the chronic diseases that plague our country.

Differences in disease expression by particular groups of patients require new designs and analyses of clinical trials, and also new approaches to validating markers or tests so that they may be useful for selecting the correct treatment for a particular person. Presently, the gold standard for clinical trials is the "randomized controlled trial" (RCT), which determines the effectiveness of a particular type of medical intervention for a specific group of patients. RCTs are discussed in Chapter 8. Criteria for eligibility and recruitment of these patients need to be stringent for the inclusion of specific groups of patients, but we should also include the largest group of similar patients for analysis. The more patients analyzed, the more statistically sound the results are that show a significant effect or benefit of a new treatment. In addition, most RCTs have patients randomly allocated to receive one or another of the treatments to be studied or an alternate control treatment or standard of care treatment. This comparison tells us if the new treatment being tested is better, worse, or no different from the control treatment. If we are to personalize medicine for an individual or a very small group of select patients, then we cannot be sure if the selection process will be objective for what we are testing. We may not have a large enough group of patients to determine statistical significance, or the test group will be too small to make the results applicable to other patients. These issues make clinical trials for personalized medical therapies difficult to validate, unless we devise better biostatistics/bioinformational methods for personalized medicine.

Another recent issue that has arisen in science and medicine is the placebo effect, which can influence clinical outcomes and treatments in approximately 40% of the population, depending on the disease. The placebo effect may call into question some of the results of RCTs and other clinical trials for pharmaceutical efficacy. This fascinating topic will be discussed in Chapter 6 and is still being actively investigated since we do not know conclusively how it will impact treatment outcomes and the delivery of healthcare. Due to placebo effects, the patient–doctor relationship grows in importance and can impact whether a patient improves in health or not. It should also be obvious from the list of medical and scientific topics discussed above that we need our doctors to help us navigate a personalized medical system. Our doctors are also needed to educate us on what therapies may be effective for our disease or for maintaining our health as we age.

There are other important topics to discuss in a book on personalized medicine, such as the costs for some of these personalized tests and therapeutics for disease and health maintenance. Can our healthcare system afford the cost? Can we develop cheaper and just as effective tests? Who should be determining the price for these tests? Which types of preventative treatments, medical procedures, and lifestyle changes are important for health? Major changes to our lifestyle appear to be absolute requirements for us to improve the health of our population. How can we enact these changes and still maintain our individual freedoms, or has our population passed the point at which we can afford total freedom? What types of changes in medical education and training need to be made in order to address this shift in medical approach for patients? Other critical topics are privacy issues and data protection. These issues will be discussed since they dramatically impact our medical system and the quality of our healthcare. In addition, if we are to personalize medicine, then we need to get used to the idea of listening to personal stories to help determine the best course for medicine. Therefore, this book is written containing individual true stories of patients and scientific advancement.

Please remember that this book is not an exhaustive analysis of personalized medicine or the complete science behind it and is colored by my own personal experiences in a healthcare center of medicine, education, and research. Rather, this book is intended to start the discussion on personalized medicine.

REFERENCES

Fuller, W. 2003. Who said 'helix'? *Nature* 424:876–8.

Jia, G, Y Fu, X Zhao et al. 2011. N6-methyladenosine in nuclear RNA is a major substrate of the obesity-associated FTO. *Nat Chem Biol* 7(12):885–7.

Tripp, S and M Grueber. 2011. *Economic Impact of the Human Genome Project*. Battelle Memorial Institute Technology.

Wang, X, Z Lu, A Gomez et al. 2014. N6-methyladenosine-dependent regulation of messenger RNA stability. *Nature* 505:117–20.

Yadav, SP. 2007. The wholeness in suffix -omics, -omes, and the word om. *J Biomol Tech* 18(5):277.

1

Genomics

Is the expression of our genes too complicated to allow us to use genomics successfully in personalized medicine?

Take a look at Figure 1.1 of the famous double helix of DNA, which will be the basis for our discussion of what genomics can and cannot do for us, as we personalize medicine.

DNA

We will start with a very short course in basic biology to introduce the terms, concepts, and essential facts for understanding genomics. The general structure of DNA is shown in Figure 1.1. Each little sphere in the picture of DNA represents a different chemical element in the DNA: carbon, oxygen, phosphorus, and nitrogen. They link together similarly to beads in order to form different compounds such as pyrimidine and purines, which spiral around each other to form the double helix. DNA is like a spiraling ladder, with specific bases paired on either side of the ladder. This structure of DNA was the famous discovery of Watson, Crick, and Wilkins, for which they received the Nobel Prize. Our genes are composed of DNA, which stores long-term instructions/sequences for the development of all of our cells into a human being. The genes are stored in the nucleus of every cell in the body. The instructions or code in the DNA are also needed to construct other components of cells, such as proteins and RNA.

Cells have two nucleic acids—DNA and RNA—which are polymers composed of monomer units that form a chain varying in length from tens to thousands of units for RNA to millions of units for DNA. The particular configuration of these components is the code for our inheritance and our proteins. Figure 1.2 shows RNA and DNA and their differences. RNA is quite similar to DNA in its structure, forming double-stranded or single-stranded linear or circular molecules with sugars and paired bases. The nucleotides of DNA and RNA are composed of a phosphate group, a pentose (a five-carbon sugar molecule), and an organic base. Nucleotides are simple building blocks for nucleic acids, in this case DNA and RNA. RNA's sugar component is a ribose. In DNA, the sugar in its structure is deoxyribose. RNA and DNA also differ in one of their bases. The bases are adenine (A), guanine (G), and cytosine (C) for both RNA and DNA, while thymidine (T) is found only in DNA and uracil (U) is found only in RNA. There are five bases: two purines, having a pair of fused ring structures—A and G—and three pyrimidines, having only one ring—C, T, and U. To form a nucleotide, each base is linked to a sugar, which can be either ribose (in the case of A, G, C, and U in RNA) or deoxyribose (for A, G, C, and T in DNA). The sugar is linked to a phosphate group. Each base is paired by hydrogen bonding to a specific base, such as A to T on either side of the DNA ladder, or C to G, etc., all the way up the sides of the DNA ladder, creating a code of bases in nucleotides. The major function of DNA is to encode the genes, which are specific sequences of bases in the DNA, along with specific RNAs that code for a protein or for another specific RNA chain. Genes hold the information to build and maintain cells, and they also pass genetic traits to the next generation through the code (for example, ACG or TGG). One side of the DNA ladder/code is copied into a complementary RNA strand and then that RNA is used to direct protein synthesis from the DNA code. Thus, the major function of RNA is protein synthesis in the cell. RNA can also act similarly to an enzyme and speed up reactions. Other RNAs found in viruses act as their genetic material instead of DNA.

CHROMOSOMES

A chromosome is an organized structure of DNA and RNA found in the nucleus of cells that contains our genes for the many different types of proteins in our body. Chromosomes also contain proteins, which package the DNA and control its function. Human beings have 46 chromosomes in each cell's nucleus (2 sets of 23 chromosomes, and therefore are diploid). The exception is the sperm and egg, which have 23 chromosomes each, so that when they combine, they form the full 46 chromosomes, similar to a book with all of the information necessary for human development.

GENES

Within the chromosome are separate units, like sentences in a book, which are genes. Genes not only encode our proteins, but also let us inherit features from our parents/ancestors. As we know, we can use different words in a sentence to express a similar meaning. In a similar manner, alleles are like different words with a different sequence in the gene that encode different effects or traits for the same feature, such as eye color. Alleles can be described as dominant or recessive. In other words, if the allele is dominant, then it will determine the appearance or function of that trait. A recessive allele will not be expressed, since the dominant allele overpowers the recessive form. However, most alleles are expressed in a more

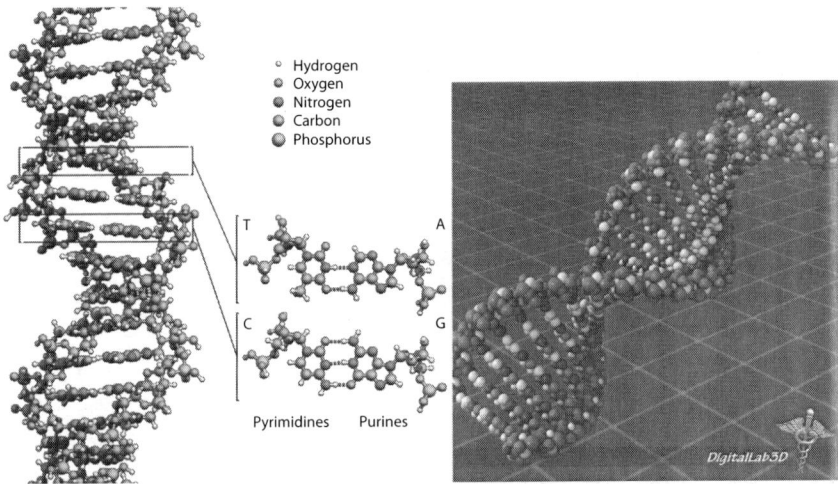

Figure 1.1 Two different representations of the double-helix structure of DNA are shown. Hydrogen, oxygen, nitrogen, carbon, and phosphorus are represented as differently colored balls, which comprise the DNA. There are four different bases that make up the "rungs" of this DNA ladder-like structure, and they are the pyrimidines—cytosine (C) and thymidine (T)—and the purines—adenine (A) and guanine (G). They are paired across the rung as either A–T or C–G. The "rails" of the ladder-like DNA structure are composed of the sugar deoxyribose and phosphate. (Reproduced with permission from Richard Wheeler. Full color version available at https://www.crcpress.com/Personalized-Medicine-Promises-and-Pitfalls/Gronowicz/9781498714914, under "Downloads/Updates".)

complicated manner than simple dominance, and many genetic variations result in little or no observable variation. Features can be physical traits such as hair or eye color, or they can be features that are not easily seen, such as blood type or a tendency for a disease. How we look, function, and express diseases is dependent on genes and the environment, including our lifestyle. Other DNA segments, besides the genes, have structural purposes or are involved in regulating the use of this genetic information. In the study of genes (genetics), the genome is an organism's hereditary information and includes genes and noncoding sequences of the DNA.

We still have much to learn about our DNA since we do not know why we have so much noncoding DNA that does not spell out an amino acid sequence for a protein. Some noncoding DNA is transcribed into functional noncoding RNA molecules, while others are not transcribed or give rise to RNAs of unknown function. The amount of noncoding DNA varies greatly among species. For example, over 98% of the human genome is noncoding DNA, while a bacterium has only 2% of its DNA as noncoding.

Chromosomal DNA encodes most of an organism's genetic information, which is copied and inherited from generation to generation. This process of inheritance involves the accurate duplication of the DNA in the cell to produce two genetically identical DNAs, and this process is called DNA replication, which is illustrated in Figure 1.3. Then the cell divides to form two identical cells with a full set of

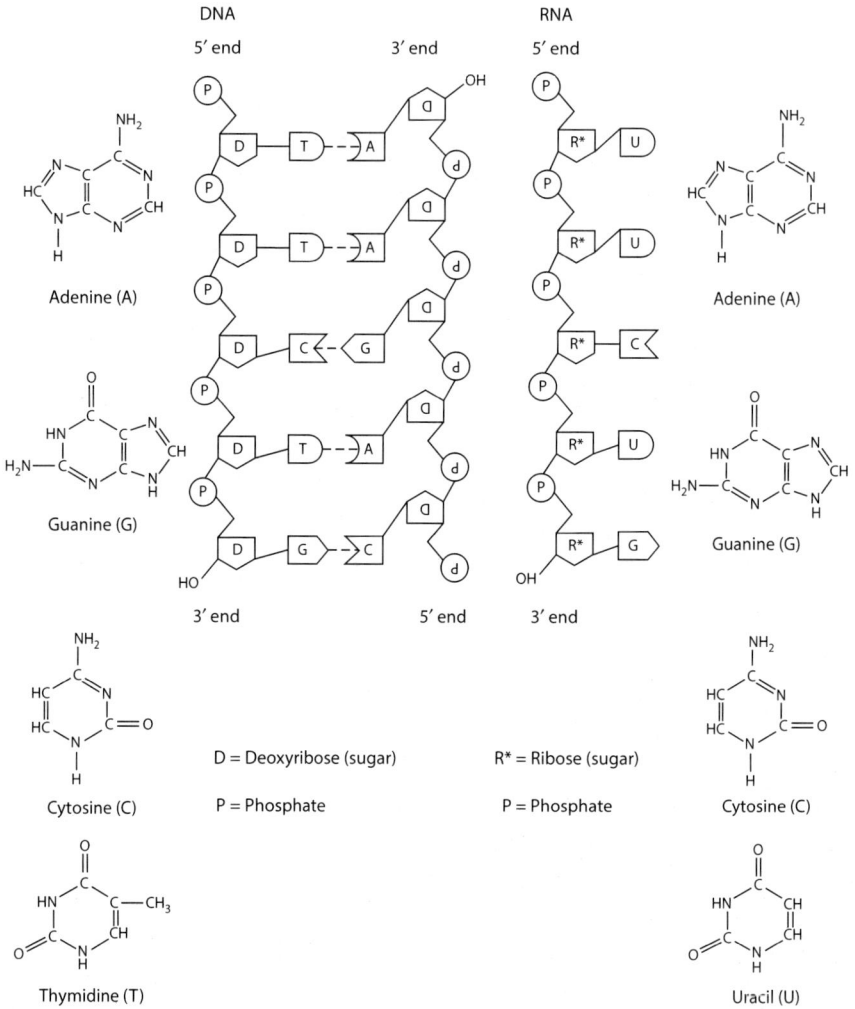

Figure 1.2 Differences between DNA and RNA. DNA is double stranded and composed of the bases adenine (A), guanine (G), cytosine (C), and thymidine (T), with their chemical compositions shown on the far left-hand side. Each base is complexed with a sugar called deoxyribose and a phosphate group to make up a nucleotide. The sugar and phosphate groups form the rail or single strand of the DNA ladder on either side. A is paired with T and C is paired with G in the ladder-like structure of DNA. The two strands of the DNA run in opposite directions to each other and are anti-parallel, running in the 5′ to 3′ direction or the 3′ to 5′ direction. RNA is usually single stranded and is composed of the bases A, G, C, and uracil (U), with their chemical compositions shown on the far right-hand side. The single backbone of the RNA is composed of nucleotides containing a particular base complexed with a phosphate group and the sugar ribose (R*).

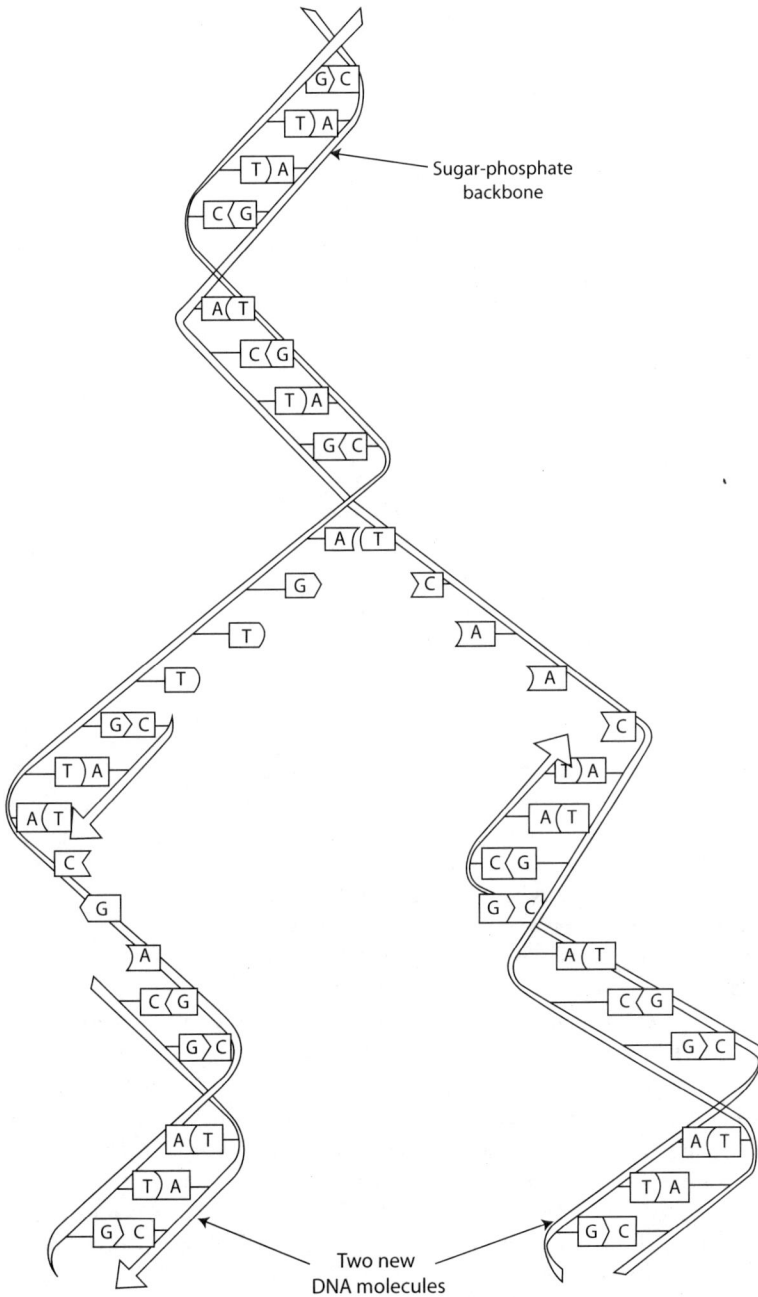

Figure 1.3 DNA replication. The ladder-like double helix of DNA is unwound and each rail carrying specific bases attached to the sugar–phosphate backbone (represented as a rail in the picture) acts as a template for creating two new double-helix DNA molecules. These two new DNA molecules are created by adding matching bases as nucleotides to the single strand.

chromosomes composed of DNA. Multiple future rounds of DNA replication creating more new cells will create tissues, and eventually create each person.

Changes in the DNA sequence can be caused by chemicals and radiation from the environment, from temperature or from reactive molecules in the cell. Therefore, there is continued surveillance and repair of the DNA due to repeated damage. A mutation is a DNA sequence that has been permanently changed (i.e., a different sequence of bases or just one base). Occasional mutations in DNA sequences can provide genetic diversity if the mutation does not have severe consequences. Some of these mutations may allow the organism to survive in changing environments and thus provide a new evolutionary step for the organism. Other mutations are harmful to the organism and can cause a particular disease or malfunction that can affect function and lifespan.

A recent exciting example of a mutation was found in a 32-year-old aerobics instructor in the Dallas, Texas area. She is healthy and has two children. Her cholesterol level is incredibly low (Kolata 2013). A rare gene mutation inherited from both her mother and father caused her to express low cholesterol levels, especially low-density lipoproteins (LDLs). Only one other person in the world—a woman from Zimbabwe—had ever been found with a comparably low level. With the identification of this rare beneficial mutation in the PCSK9 gene, numerous drug companies are in a race to find a drug that can mimic this DNA mutation to decrease LDL levels, which, perhaps, can prevent heart attacks.

TRANSCRIPTION AND TRANSLATION

Genetic information is expressed in cells by the mechanisms of transcription and translation. The DNA in the chromosomes of the genome does not directly carry out protein synthesis, but uses RNA as an intermediary. The DNA is like the board of directors of a company that uses employees—the RNA—to carry out its directives. These directives form a process called transcription in which particular DNA/nucleotide sequences are copied into RNA. One side of the DNA ladder/code is copied into a complementary RNA strand with complementary nucleotides. Then that RNA, called messenger RNA (mRNA), is used to direct protein synthesis from the DNA code. This mRNA is used as a template to direct the synthesis of a particular protein in a process called translation. Figure 1.4 illustrates transcription and translation.

The final RNA product is created by splicing to remove introns—any nucleotide sequence within a gene—and joining the exons—the nucleotide sequences that remain after splicing. Introns are found in the genes of most organisms and many viruses, and can be located in a wide range of genes, including those that generate proteins, ribosomal RNA (rRNA), and transfer RNA (tRNA). When

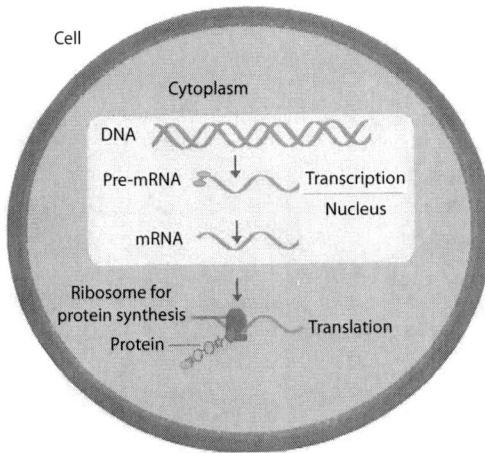

Figure 1.4 Transcription and translation. A diagram of a cell with its central nucleus and surrounding cytoplasm is shown. In the nucleus, transcription takes place. The DNA unwinds and one strand of the DNA is transcribed into an RNA molecule, with additional enzymes and proteins participating in the process to help encode at least one gene. If the gene that is transcribed is a particular protein, then messenger RNA (mRNA) will be created with the appropriate nucleotides for encoding that protein. The mRNA is transcribed as a more complex RNA or pre-RNA, with exons and introns and other modifications there to direct its fate. Introns are removed by RNA splicing so that the exons remain to be covalently joined in order to create the mature mRNA that encodes the protein. The mRNA leaves the nucleus and enters the cytoplasm, where it will be translated into a protein while attached to a ribosome. A ribosome is a large and complex machine of proteins and enzymes involved in the process of translation for making a protein composed of amino acids as determined by the particular mRNA code.

proteins are generated from intron-containing genes, RNA splicing occurs in the RNA processing pathway that follows transcription and precedes translation.

THE BIRTH OF GENETICS AND MENDEL

With the basic knowledge of genes, DNA and the processes of DNA replication, transcription, and translation, we can move onto seeing how these biological processes contribute to the personal genetics of each person and also to their family history. The more simple form of inheritance is Mendelian genetics or monogenetics. Gregor Johann Mendel was a friar and a scientist who lived in the nineteenth century. He studied the inheritance of various characteristics of pea plants—seed shape, flower color, seed coat color, shape, and color of ripe and unripe pods, flower location, and plant height—that he could observe growing at his monastery. He demonstrated that these traits follow particular patterns, now referred to as Mendelian inheritance. Between 1856 and 1863,

Mendel studied some 29,000 pea plants and showed that one in four plants had purebred recessive alleles, two out of four were hybrid, and one out of four were purebred dominant. From this work, he developed the Law of Segregation of Alleles and the Law of Independent Assortment, which were not accepted by the scientific community until a long time after his death. However, in the twentieth century, these laws have become the basis for modern-day genetics. An allele is one of a number of different forms of the same gene or same genetic locus on the chromosome. Each allele can produce different effects, as is found in eye color.

The Law of Segregation states that the two alleles for a heritable characteristic separate from each other and end up in different gametes, in our case the sperm or the egg. Interactions between alleles at a single locus can influence how the offspring expresses that trait (dominance of one allele over another recessive allele will determine the outcome). The Law of Independent Assortment states that separate genes for separate traits are passed independently of one another from parents to offspring. For example, seed shape would be inherited independently of plant height. From these principles defined by Mendel and his seemingly simple experiments with almost 30,000 plants, we can now demonstrate that some of our human diseases are inherited in the same manner. So the study of plants helped us understand ourselves, and shows that we are all connected by basic principles in science.

Marfan Syndrome and Mendelian Genetics

Marfan syndrome is a disease that follows Mendelian genetics. People with Marfan syndrome are unusually tall with long limbs and fingers. The disease is caused by misfolding of the protein fibrillin-1. Fibrillin-1 binds to itself to form thread-like filaments called microfibrils, which form elastic fibers. In connective tissues, elastic fibers allow the skin, ligaments, and blood vessels to stretch. Connective tissue is a tissue in our bodies that supports, connects, or separates different types of tissues and organs. There is connective tissue around each of our organs and it is found everywhere in the body except the central nervous system. Fibrillin is encoded by the gene FBN1, which is recessive or not apparently expressed (Kainulainen et al. 1994; Dietz et al. 2005). If a person inherits one copy of the MarfanFBN1 gene from both parents, thereby having two MarfanFBN1 genes, then he/she will develop Marfan syndrome. Patients with Marfan syndrome can have mild to severe disease expression, with the most serious complications causing defects in the heart valves and aorta, which can result in aortic aneurysms and death. Additionally, it may affect the lungs, eyes, spinal cord, skeleton, and hard palate in the mouth. With the knowledge of the genetics of its inheritance and the gene responsible for this disease, doctors have been able to intervene in the disease and prevent early death.

However, in general, genetics is not simple for most traits and diseases. This complexity and the cost required in order to understand genomics may become a pitfall in genomics unless we creatively solve these issues. Without a thorough understanding of genomics, we cannot decide whether this approach will improve medicine or cause increased costs without significant benefit to our medical system and health.

MITOSIS, MEIOSIS, AND RECOMBINATION

To start explaining the complexity of gene expression, the processes of mitosis, meiosis, and genetic recombination will be described. Within normal tissues, cells duplicate their chromosomes and divide (replicate) by a process called mitosis in order to make two cells from one parent cell. Each cell has a complete set of chromosomes. Mitosis increases the number of cells in that tissue. During mitosis, recombination is a rare occurrence. Once chromosomes are duplicated, the two homologous chromosomes are next to each other and can overlap. In the process of overlapping, a double-stranded break can occur in both homologous chromosomes. This break is then repaired by having the two broken parts join with the homologous chromosome partner in order to reform in a process called recombination. Recombination that occurs between two sister chromosomes derived from duplication of the original DNA strand often does not result in rearrangement of the genes, since these sister chromosomes are usually identical or homologous. Recombination is more common in meiosis.

During the process of meiosis, the 46 chromosomes are halved to form two gametes, in our case the egg or the sperm, each containing 23 chromosomes. Non-sister chromosomes can pair with each other, and if recombination occurs from one strand of DNA to the other non-sister DNA, then new combinations of alleles occur, resulting in a rearrangement of genes. Figure 1.5 illustrates the processes

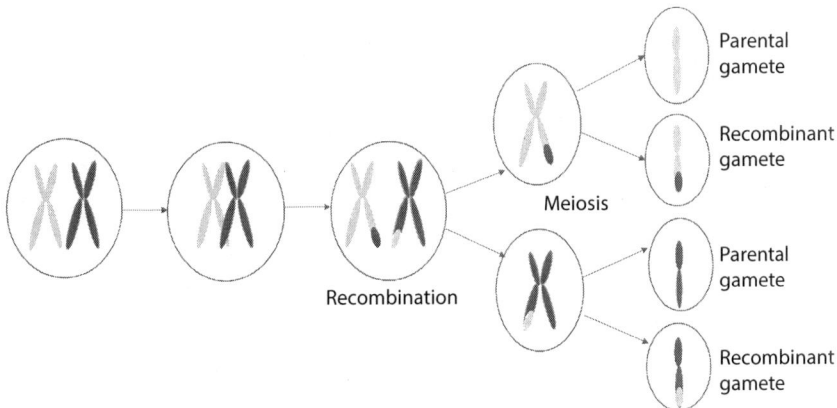

Figure 1.5 Recombination in meiosis. Recombination occurs when two different or non-sister chromosomes, illustrated as gray and black, break their DNA and then recombine to form a new combination of alleles. During meiosis, when these altered chromosomes are segregated into the sperm and the egg forming a recombinant gamete, this new pattern for inheritance, illustrated as a combination of gray and black, is then passed down to the progeny. In this manner, the progeny acquires a different combination of alleles in order to make them unique.

of meiosis and recombination. Upon fertilization with the fusion of sperm and egg, the number of sets of chromosomes is restored to 46 chromosomes, but with unique rearrangements of the genes to create a new individual. For example, sperm contains 23 chromosomes, and the possible number of different sperm cells based on different chromosome combinations is $2^{23} = 8,388,608$. This complexity of inheritance can explain some of the reasons why we may look so different from our parents. It is this diversity that can help us to survive changing environments, cause us to lose a baby in utero, or cause a disease. Recombination makes it is difficult to determine the origin of a person's genes that may cause a disease or improve the health status of an individual. Where and when did the change occur in the DNA? Therefore, is the tendency for a particular disease due to inheritance or another reason?

SINGLE-NUCLEOTIDE POLYMORPHISM

The variations in our DNA that can occur at the single-nucleotide level are called single-nucleotide polymorphisms (SNPs), with "SNP" being pronounced "snip." These SNPs can be found between paired chromosomes of different biological species or human beings. For example, one DNA has ACTTGA, while the other paired chromosome has ACTTAA, which vary in one SNP, as shown in Figure 1.6. If we consider the DNA as a language with different words representing each gene, then a SNP is a change in a letter of that word. Most SNPs occur in noncoding regions rather than the coding regions of our genes. Factors such as genetic recombination and mutation rate can determine how many SNPs are found in particular regions of the DNA. These variations in DNA

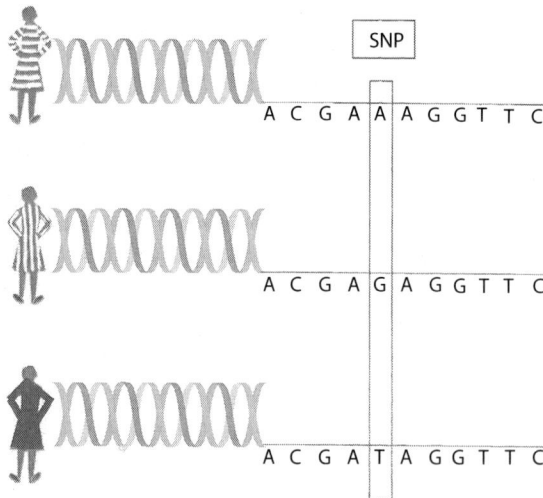

Figure 1.6 Single-nucleotide polymorphism (SNP). A SNP is a variation in the DNA sequence in which a single nucleotide is changed. In the illustrated case, it is an A which is changed to a G or a T in the genome, so that the individuals shown have different alleles that encode different characteristic traits.

sequences may be the cause of a disease or affect our responses to chemicals, drugs, and even vaccines. Thus, SNPs are an important part of personalized medicine. In genome-wide association study (GWAS) between groups of people with or without a disease, we hope to be able to determine which SNPs in a particular gene may contribute to that disease. Both cystic fibrosis and sickle-cell anemia have been shown to have SNPs in specific genes that contribute to disease manifestation (Ingram 1956; Hamosh et al. 1992; Gisler et al. 2013).

SNPs can also be used for practical purposes, such as in forensic science, in which genetic variations in SNPs between individuals can be used for DNA fingerprinting. That is why forensic experts can be so sure of their results linking a person to a crime because the total length of the human genome is over 3 billion base pairs. If a fingerprint displays particular sequences of SNPs and these are found in a particular chromosome, then a suspect can be identified from a sample of their DNA.

An issue with SNPs is that, in many diseases, SNPs do not function individually; rather, a group of SNPs works together to manifest a disease, so it becomes very complicated to understand the cause of a disease. As of 2013, 62,676,337 SNPs have been found in humans (National Center for Biotechnology Information 2013). The diversity of our genes is amazing and also shows us how complicated human biology can be with all of these SNPs. It becomes difficult to understand completely a disease or our physiology, which is the expression of all of these factors.

Osteoporosis and SNPs

An example of a disease that has many SNPs contributing to its expression is osteoporosis (Singh et al. 2010). Osteoporosis is a skeletal disease characterized by low bone mass and deterioration of bone microstructure, leading to an increased rate of fracture. Deterioration of the bone structure leading to osteoporotic bone fractures is shown in Figure 1.7. It is a global health concern since

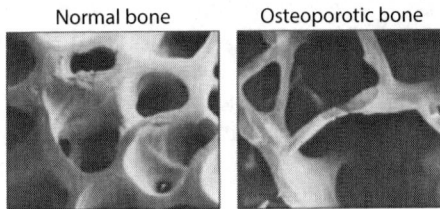

Figure 1.7 Normal and osteoporotic bone with a fracture from human biopsies, as seen in scanning electron micrographs. Normal bone is shown on the left with a honeycomb-like structure, in which the bone plates are interconnected. In the right-hand panel, osteoporotic bone is shown with thinner plates that appear more like rods that are weaker and most susceptible to fracture. In the middle is a fracture in which the rod-like structure of bone is broken. (Reproduced from Dempster, DW et al., *J Bone Miner Res.* 1986; 1(1):15–21, with permission from the American Society of Bone and Mineral Research.)

osteoporosis results in approximately 9 million fractures per year and it has been estimated that approximately half of all women and a quarter of men over the age of 50 in the United States will experience a hip fracture in their lifetime (Johnell and Kanis 2006; Nguyen et al. 2007).

Measuring bone mineral density (BMD) helps to determine the risk for osteoporosis and assess if there is a need for drugs and/or other therapeutic modalities that would prevent further bone loss and possible fractures. BMD is the amount of mineral per square centimeter of bone. Most often, doctors use an instrument to scan the lumber hip and spine with low radiation (dual x-ray absorptiometry [DXA]) in order to determine BMD. However, DXA is not highly sensitive in predicting fracture risk in an individual, but rather gives us guidelines for the population as a whole and screens individuals for therapeutic intervention (Mitchell and Streeten 2013). The Fracture Risk Assessment Tool (FRAX®) was developed in order to improve diagnosis by also considering gender, height, weight, prior fragility fracture, parental history of hip fracture, rheumatoid arthritis, use of oral glucocorticoids, and behavioral factors, such as smoking and alcohol consumption of three or more units daily, as risk factors in the 10-year probability of a major osteoporotic fracture (Kanis et al. 2009). Again, our behaviors can influence our ability to express a disease. Interestingly, increased body weight is consistently associated with a higher BMD, lower hip fracture rate, and reduced likelihood of osteoporosis.

Bone is dynamic in that it is continually being formed and resorbed during a person's lifetime, and the peak bone mass gained in the first 25 years of life is critical as to whether a person becomes osteoporotic as they age. For everyone, peak bone mass is obtained in the early 20s, maintained until the 30s and 40s, and followed by a slow decline with age, but accelerates greatly in women during menopause. A graph of the changes in peak bone mass for men and women is shown in Figure 1.8. Peak bone mass is also greatly affected by early nutrition and lifestyle factors, and some doctors consider osteoporosis as an adult disease with "its seeds in childhood" (Mitchell and Streeten 2013). These facts support the importance of athletic programs in school and out of school, so that boys and especially girls exercise and increase bone mass in their early years (Kemmler et al. 2015). We can think of this issue as having a half-empty glass for bone mass. If your glass is half full at the start of the day, then you will get to the bottom of the glass sooner than if you started with a full glass (i.e., bone mass). In addition, low bone mass in aging adults increases mortality with fractures, and there is a decrease in the quality of life, often due to chronic pain, functional limitations, and psychological issues.

An example is my mother who, at the age of 82, fell in her home where she lived by herself, and suffered a small crack in her hip. She was diagnosed with osteoporosis at that time and told to take it easy at home. Nothing could be done medically except for physical therapy for a few months. Her whole life changed because of her own attitude about her health, a fear of falling again, and lack of physical activity. After taking it easy for several weeks, she had weakened considerably. She stopped her avid gardening, and with time became more reclusive and more negative about life. She sold her house and moved into an independent assisted-living facility. I saw her change from a witty, vibrant woman into a negative and fearful person that started with her small fracture. My mother is not an isolated case in the elderly population, because a fracture of the hip often has a snowball effect, causing more and more physical and mental health problems. She was lucky in that she did not break her hip, which results in excess mortality of 18% within the first 6 months (Tosteson et al. 2007).

Although we do not know the causes of osteoporosis, family history contributes strongly to BMD, with genes contributing 60%–80% of the variability in BMD. Therefore, there is considerable research into which genes may be responsible (Peacock et al. 2002; Ng et al. 2006). Numerous GWAS have been performed in order to test the hypothesis that there is an association of genetic differences in the population with a minor allele frequency. The largest GWAS study of BMD was undertaken by the Genetic Factors of Osteoporosis Consortium with 32,000 subjects (Estrada et al. 2012) and determined that there were 56 loci associated with BMD, of which 14 loci were associated with fracture. Each of these 14 loci's contribution to fracture rates was very small, accounting together for far less than 1% of BMD. With all of the loci considered

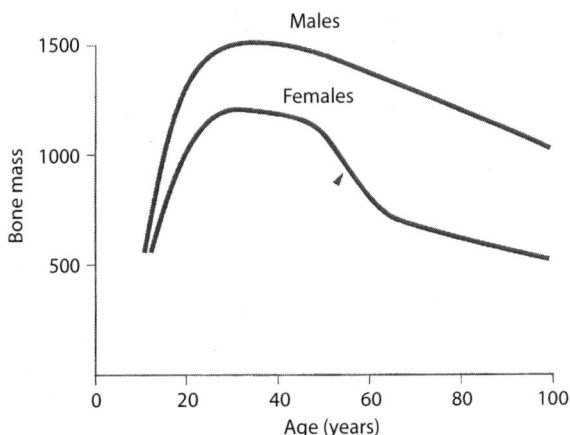

Figure 1.8 Average bone loss with age. In the first 25 years in the lives of both males (top line) and females (bottom line), there is rapid bone growth, with males reaching a higher bone mass than women in their 30s. Then, both groups start to lose bone with age. However, at menopause (approximately 50+ years; see arrowhead), women have a more precipitous drop in bone mass. In their 60+ years, both males and females lose bone mass at the same rate.

together, the contribution to fracture rate was only approximately 5% of BMD. More GWAS are being published each year by this group, but these SNPs have an even smaller effect size and cannot predict a person's risk of fracture. Therefore, genomics has been unable to discover the genes that are most responsible for BMD, osteoporosis, or bone fractures so far. Different groups of scientists are actively debating the value of genomics and personalized medicine for contributing essential information regarding our chronic diseases, such as osteoporosis, which appear to be too complicated in their expression for us to determine which genetic components and/or environmental factors contribute most to maintaining bone mass with age and avoiding osteoporosis at this point in time (Nebert and Zhang 2012).

However, one goal of the GWAS, which may be attainable, is to obtain information on specific genes in a disease pathway that can help us understand the pathology of that disease. With this information, drug therapy may be developed for targeting this specific disease pathway (Mitchell and Streeten 2013). However, the dream of finding the key to osteoporosis and fracture risk still remains elusive with the genomics approach, and may not be attainable unless new technical and scientific discoveries are made in this line of research.

CYSTIC FIBROSIS, CANCER, AND GENOMICS

In personalized medicine, the genomic approach may be more successful in determining the cause of a disease that affects a smaller group of patients and has fewer genes associated with disease expression or phenotype. In such a case, we might have a better chance of using genomics to produce a novel therapy to help a particular group of patients. Cystic fibrosis (CF) is technically a rare disease, but it is the most widespread life-shortening genetic disease that affects mostly people of Central and Northern European ancestry, with approximately 30,000 people in the United States having the disease. CF is caused by a mutation in the gene for the protein cystic fibrosis transmembrane conductance regulator (CFTR), which is unable to function in these CF patients. The cause of the disease is abnormal transport of chloride and sodium across the epithelium—the layer of cells that line the surfaces of our bodies and also line hollow organs and glands. The disease affects the lungs, pancreas, liver, and intestines, but it is the changes in the lungs and inability to breathe that cause such terrible problems for the patient. It is a recessive disease in that it requires both the mother and father to contribute their mutated CFTR gene in order for a child to develop cystic fibrosis. The variability in severity of disease expression has recently been discovered to be due to SNPs in genes that code for proteins that interact with CFTR protein expression, trafficking to the cell membrane, and function. These SNPs were correlated with various lung functions in the patients from whom these genetic analyses were made (Gisler et al. 2013). Thus, disease severity in CF is modified by other genes with different SNPs that interact with CFTR. Knowledge of SNPs increases our understanding of the activities of CFTR in cells and helps explain why disease severity differs among patients. It is hoped that this knowledge will lead to new therapeutics.

A pitfall for personalized medicine can be found in the cost of the drug Kalydeco from Vertex. This drug works very well for the 2200 world-wide CF patients who have a particular mutation, called G551D, and prolongs their lives. The cost is $307,000 per year per patient (Herper 2014). Recently, a combination of Kalydeco and the drug Lumacaftor has been introduced. This may help more patients—approximately 22,000 people over the age of 12 in the United States—but not as efficiently in terms of lung capacity as Kalydeco. The combination drug will cost approximately $160,000 per year per patient. The question for our medical care system is: how can we sustain these types of pharmaceutical costs as more designer drugs are developed for personalized medicine? On the other hand, for families who have a child with CF, they want that child to have a normal, full life. Our medical system has to be ready for these challenges and be able to solve them in a more humane and cost-effective way.

POST-TRANSLATIONAL MODIFICATIONS

However, as we can see from examples of various diseases, simple cataloging of genomic mutations and rearrangements is not enough to explain the complex cellular processes involved in the expression of a particular protein, or even more complex cellular processes such as cell growth and death, cell differentiation into mature cell types, or aging with changes in a multitude of proteins. Then there are different rates of degradation of proteins and RNAs, which affect how proteins will be expressed. When we combine genomics and proteomics, in general, the level of transcription of a gene gives only a very rough estimate of its level of translation into a protein. The reason for this is that many transcripts of a particular gene can produce more than one protein through splicing and post-translational modifications (Figure 2.1; and see Chapter 2 for a more thorough description of post-translational modifications). Alternative splicing is a process of gene expression in which particular regions of a gene may be included or excluded from the final mRNA so that different proteins are produced. Alternative splicing produces more proteins than would be expected from about 20,000 protein-coding genes of the human genome. Post-translational modifications also create different functioning proteins, but not through the genes. An example of a post-translational modification of a protein is phosphorylation—the addition of a phosphate group to a protein, which then changes its function. One of the most important examples of phosphorylation is in maintaining our body's water content through the phosphorylation of sodium/phosphate-adenosine triphosphatase (ATPase). Sodium/phosphate-ATPases mediate the transport of sodium and potassium ions across each cell's membrane in order to maintain osmoregulation—the maintenance of the proper water content in a cell—which is critical for life.

Melinda Bachini, a mother of six children, owes her continued survival of a deadly cancer called metastatic cholangiocarcinoma to a genomics approach to her cancer (Grady 2014; Tran et al. 2014). Researchers were able to identify particular immune cells that attacked a specific mutation in her malignant cells. After growing these immune cells in the laboratory, they were able to give her back these immune cells, which caused shrinkage of her tumors. Melinda is not completely cured, but she is continuing to survive a disease that would have taken her life in a few months. The hope for the future is to harness a person's immune system to fight cancer with the use of genomic techniques.

MICROARRAYS AND CRISPR/CAS9

Many different methods have been developed for the detection of specific genes. Microarrays are widely used for genes and other biological factors. They are two-dimensional maps or chips consisting of large numbers of genes or proteins on a solid substrate such as a glass slide or silicon thin-film that are used for the screening and detection of specific sequences. Microarrays allow for high-throughput, multiplexed, and parallel screening of many biological factors using identical methods in order to identity and quantity specific genes, proteins, or other factors. Microarrays have been developed for DNA, microRNA, protein, chemical compounds, carbohydrates, and materials. However, the microarray was first developed for antibodies by Tse Wen Chang (1983). The development of a quantitative technique for monitoring gene expression by microarray created the "gene chip" industry (Schena et al. 1995).

Briefly, the basic technique for a microarray is as follows: each spot on the solid substrate, such as a glass plate, contains picomoles (10^{-12} moles) of a specific DNA sequence, known as a probe (or a reporter or oligo). They can be a short sequence of a gene or other DNA element. Thus, one needs to have sequenced the genomes and created specific probes for specific genes of interest, and attached them onto the substrate. These microarrays are what are created and marketed by different companies. Alternatively, these microarrays with specific probes can be synthesized by a laboratory for its own use. The probes are then hybridized to a complementary DNA (cDNA) or a cRNA under high-stringency conditions so as to allow for specific and strong binding. The cDNA or cRNA is produced from the sample of interest, perhaps from a single individual, cell, or tissue sample. Hybridization is usually detected and quantified by fluorescent markers (fluorophore-), silver-, or chemiluminescent-labeled targets in order to determine the relative abundance of the specific DNA sequence or genes of interest. High standards must be maintained in order to produce scientifically valuable and consistent results. The first replication of the biological sample of interest is critical to carrying conclusions from one experiment to another. Second, technical replicates, (i.e., replicates of the same extraction) have to be made in order to ensure reproducibility of the findings. Finally, there have to be replicates of the probes on the same glass slide in order to ensure that hybridization and target detection are consistent. Statistical arrays of the large data sets that are generated from microarray results must also be made, and these need to take into account background noise. Normalization of the data with specific standards is also required.

Microarrays have become a common technique and have allowed scientists to screen gene expression more quickly in their biological systems and/or a patient's gene expression in a particular tissue. An exciting example of the use of microarrays has been the development of microarrays to screen one drop of a person's blood in order to determine every virus to which the person has ever been exposed (Xu et al. 2015). The microarray detects antibodies—the specific proteins made by the immune system that are produced in response to any virus. This test can be performed in the laboratory for as little as $25. Although not perfect, this method represents a novel and major step forward in the comprehensive analysis of what an individual may have been exposed to in his/her lifetime. This test may help doctors to understand the etiology of a disease.

A relatively new method for gene editing—adding or deleting genes—is clustered regularly interspaced short palindromic repeats (CRISPR)/CRISPR-associated protein 9 (Cas9). This is a bacteria-derived system that uses RNA to recognize specific human DNA sequences and then uses an endonuclease—Cas9—to cut the required sequence for genetic manipulation. CRISPRs themselves are segments of bacterial DNA that contain short repetitious base sequences. Each repetition has even shorter spacer DNA segments that are created from previous exposure of the bacterium to a virus or plasmid. By delivering Cas9 and appropriate guide RNAs in order to recognize a particular sequence, an organism's genome can be cut at any desired location and a gene either removed or added (Chapter 11 further describes this new technology).

CHIMERA

To complicate further the field of genomics, scientists are finding that there can be multiple genomes within one individual, which may not be as uncommon as was once thought. Twins can have a mixture of their genomes through sharing blood vessels in the womb, or two fertilized eggs may fuse and become an embryonic chimera, which develops into one human being (Chen et al. 2013). The word "chimera" is derived from Greek mythology, in which a chimera was a fire-breathing monster with a lion's head, a goat's body, and a serpent's tail. In biology, a chimera is a single organism composed of genetically distinct cells. Women can also gain genomes from their children by a process in which fetal cells remain in the mother's body, where they can travel to different organs and colonize those tissues. Scientists are beginning to find that multiple genomes can be linked to some rare diseases, such as some autoimmune thyroid diseases, specifically Hashimoto thyroiditis and Graves' disease. However, more common instances of mosaicism seem to be normal for human tissues (O'Huallachain 2012). The extent of chimeras in human physiology will have to be taken into consideration as genomics becomes the basis of personalized medicine.

Scientists will forever continue to learn about the complex patterns of gene and protein expression. These patterns create the many cellular processes of cells and tissues, and changes to these patterns can lead to disease. The idea of being able to personalize diagnosis and treatment for each person, which we see promised by medical institutions and groups of doctors, seems at this point beyond our reach for the majority of patients. Is it worth striving for? I believe it is, because we are learning more and more about normal cellular processes and diseases, but patients should know that we are far from achieving this goal of personalized medicine due to the complexity of each person's physiology. For a few individuals, such as Melinda Bachini, this hope has become a reality.

REFERENCES

Chang, T-W. 1983. Binding of cells to matrixes of distinct antibodies coated on solid surface. *J Immunol Methods* 65(1–2):217–23.

Chen, K, RH Chmait, D Vanderbilt, S Wu, and L Randolph. 2013. Chimerism in monochorionic dizygotic twins: Case study and review. *Am J Med Genet Part A* 161A:1817–24.

Dietz, HC, B Loeys, L Carta, and F Ramirez. 2005. Recent progress towards a molecular understanding of Marfan syndrome. *Am J Med Genet C Semin Med Genet* 139C(1):4–9.

Estrada, K, U Styrkarsdottir, E Evangelou et al. 2012. Genome-wide meta-analysis identifies 56 bone mineral density loci and reveals 14 loci associated with risk of fracture. *Nat Genet* 44(5):491–501.

Gisler, FM, T von Kanel, R Kraemer, A Schaller, and S Gallati. 2013. Identification of SNPs in the cystic fibrosis interactome influencing pulmonary progression in cystic fibrosis. *Eur J Hum Genet* 21(4):397–403.

Grady, D. 2014. Patient's cells deployed to attack aggressive cancer. *NY Times* May 9:A3.

Hamosh, A, TM King, BJ Rosenstein et al. 1992. Cystic fibrosis patients bearing both the common missense mutation Gly–Asp at codon 551 and the delta F508 mutation are clinically indistinguishable from delta F508 homozygotes, except for decreased risk of meconium ileus. *Am J Hum Genet* 51(2):245–50.

Herper, M. 2014. In a victory for gene research, Vertex drug combo clears lungs clogged by cystic fibrosis. *Forbes-Pharma and Healthcare* no. 6/24/2014: http://www.forbes.com/sites/matthewherper/2014/06/24/in-a-victory-for-gene-research-drugs-clear-lungs-clogged-by-cystic-fibrosis/

Ingram, VM. 1956. A specific chemical difference between the globins of normal human and sickle-cell anaemia haemoglobin. *Nature* 178(4537):792–4.

Johnell, O and JA Kanis. 2006. An estimate of the worldwide prevalence and disability associated with osteoporotic fractures. *Osteoporos Int* 17:1726–33.

Kainulainen, K, L Karttunen, L Puhakka, L Sakai, and L Peltonen. 1994. Mutations in the fibrillin gene responsible for dominant ectopia lentis and neonatal Marfan syndrome. *Nat Genet* 6(1):64–9.

Kanis, JA, A Oden, H Johnsson, F Borstrom, O Strom, and E McCloskey. 2009. FRAX® and its application to clinical practice. *Bone* 44:734–43.

Kemmler, W, M Bebenek, S von Stengel, and J Bauer. 2015. Peak-bone-mass development in young adults: Effects of study program related levels of occupational and leisure time physical activity and exercise. A prospective 5-year study. *Osteoporos Int* 26(2):653–62.

Kolata, G. 2013. Rare mutation ignites race for cholesterol drug. *NY Times* July 10:A1.

Mitchell, BD and EA Streeten. 2013. Clinical impact of recent genetic discoveries in osteoporosis. *Appl Clin Genet* 6:75–85.

National Center for Biotechnology Information. 2013. NCBI dbSNP build 138 for human and cow. *United States National Library of Medicine.* http://www.ncbi.nlm.nih.gov/mailman/pipermail/dbsnp-announce /2013q3/000133.html.

Nebert, DW and G Zhang. 2012. Personalized medicine: Temper expectations. *Science* 337:910–1.

Ng, MY, PC Sham, AD Patterson, V Chan, and AW Kung. 2006. Effect of environmental factors and gender on the heritability of bone mineral density and bone size. *Ann Hum Genet* 70:428–38.

Nguyen, ND, HG Ahlborg, JR Center, JA Eisman, and TV Nguyen. 2007. Residual lifetime risk of fractures in women and men. *J Bone Mineral Res* 22:781–8.

O'Huallachain M, KJ Karczewski, SM Weissman, AE Urban, and MP Snyder. 2012. Extensive genetic variation in somatic human tissues. *Proc Natl Acad Sci USA* 109(44):18018–23.

Peacock, M, CH Turner, MJ Econs, and T Foroud. 2002. Genetics of osteoporosis. *Endocr Rev* 23:303–26.

Schena, M, D Shalon, RW Davis, and PO Brown. 1995. Quantitative monitoring of gene expression patterns with a complementary DNA microarray. *Science* 270(5235):467–70.

Singh, M, P Singh, PK Juneja, S Singh, and T Kaur. 2010. SNP–SNP interactions within APOE gene influence plasma lipids in postmenopausal osteoporosis. *Rheum Int* 31(3):421–3.

Tosteson, AN, DJ Gottlieb, DC Radley, ES Fisher, and LJ Melton 3rd. 2007. Excess mortality following hip fracture: The role of underlying health status. *Osteoporos Int* 18:1463–72.

Tran, E, S Turcotte, A Gros et al. 2014. Cancer immunotherapy based on mutation-specific CD4+ T cells in a patient with epithelial cancer. *Science* 344:641–5.

Xu, GJ, Y Kula, Q Xu et al. 2015. Viral immunology. Comprehensive serological profiling of human populations using a synthetic human virome. *Science* 348(6329):aaa0698.

2

Proteomics

Can proteomics help us to diagnose and treat diseases in individuals?

Proteins/proteomics are important to personalized medicine since sick cells, cancer cells, and normal cells will express specific proteins on their surfaces and inside the cell that reflect a cell's activities and health. If a protein is specific for a cancer cell, then we can perhaps target that cell for destruction using a drug that is specific to that protein. However, if that protein produced by the cancer cell is also produced by another type of healthy cell in the body, then we may have difficulty targeting the cancer cell without hurting the healthy cell. Most chemotherapies target fast-growing cells for destruction, meaning that other healthy cells that proliferate rapidly, such as the epithelium that lines our mouth and digestive tract, our hair, and other cells in tissues, are killed. Chemotherapy has numerous side effects such as hair loss, nausea, vomiting, and neurological deficits. If we can find therapies using proteomics that target a more select group of abnormal cells, then we can more successfully rid our bodies of the disease with fewer side effects. To bring proteomic results to the clinic, we must also verify these findings discovered in the laboratory with multiple different and independent quantitative investigative procedures (assays) that support targeting of that one protein or a few proteins. Proteomic results must also be verified with an analysis of a large number of patients with that disease, and they must determine what percentage of the patients are cured after 5–10 years and what, if any, the short- and long-term side effects are of that therapy.

In proteomics, the entire set of proteins expressed by the genome in cells, tissues, and organisms is called the proteome. To study the proteome, a defined set of conditions such as developmental stage, health status, environment, etc., are required, since the proteome will change depending on conditions. In fact, the human proteome is more complex than the human genome, which is comprised of 20,000–25,000 genes. Figure 2.1 demonstrates that single genes encode multiple proteins by processes such as recombination, transcription that is initiated or terminated at different sites, and alternative splicing of the transcript in order to generate different mRNA transcripts from a single gene. However, the total number of proteins in the human proteome (Figure 2.1) is estimated at over 1 million (Jensen 2004). This complexity of the proteome is generated by

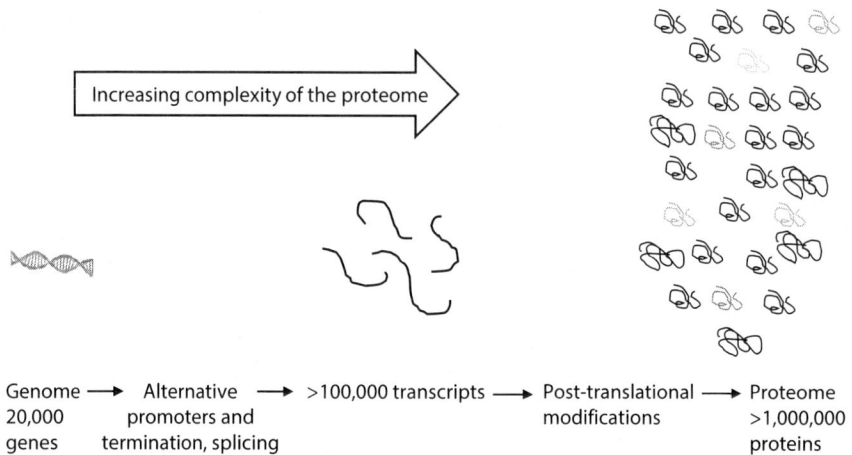

Genome → Alternative → >100,000 transcripts → Post-translational → Proteome
20,000   promoters and   modifications   >1,000,000
genes   termination, splicing   proteins

Figure 2.1 Proteome. The genome comprises about 20,000–25,000 genes, while the proteome is very complex and is estimated to have over 1 million proteins. Changes at the transcriptional and mRNA levels increase the number and diversity of transcripts. However, it is the post-translational modifications of these transcripts that exponentially increase the complexity of the proteome relative to the genome.

protein post-translational modifications, which are chemical modifications to a protein that regulate their activity, localization, and interactions with other molecules. We will briefly discuss these post-translational modifications that create the complex proteome.

AMINO ACIDS AND PROTEINS

We will start with a very short course in basic biology to introduce the terms, concepts, and essential facts for understanding proteomics. The building blocks of proteomics and the building blocks of cells in our bodies are proteins, which are composed of different amino acids. Figure 2.2 is a diagram of a generic amino acid. Table 2.1 is a list of the most common amino acids, which number 20, although there are others that are rare. We can conceive of amino acids as letters of the protein alphabet. Particular sequences of these letters/amino acids make up a particular word/protein. These amino acids are joined together in many different combinations that form long chains. In cells, typical proteins consist of 100–500 amino acids and are called polypeptides that have meaning for the human body, just like letters in particular arrangements have meaning in language. The longest known protein chain is built from more than 34,000 amino acids (titin, a protein found in muscles), similarly to one of the longest words in the English language, antidisestablishmentarianism. The amino acid chain in the protein, insulin, is shown in Figure 2.2. There are many different proteins carrying out many different functions in cells and tissues, just as each word means something different.

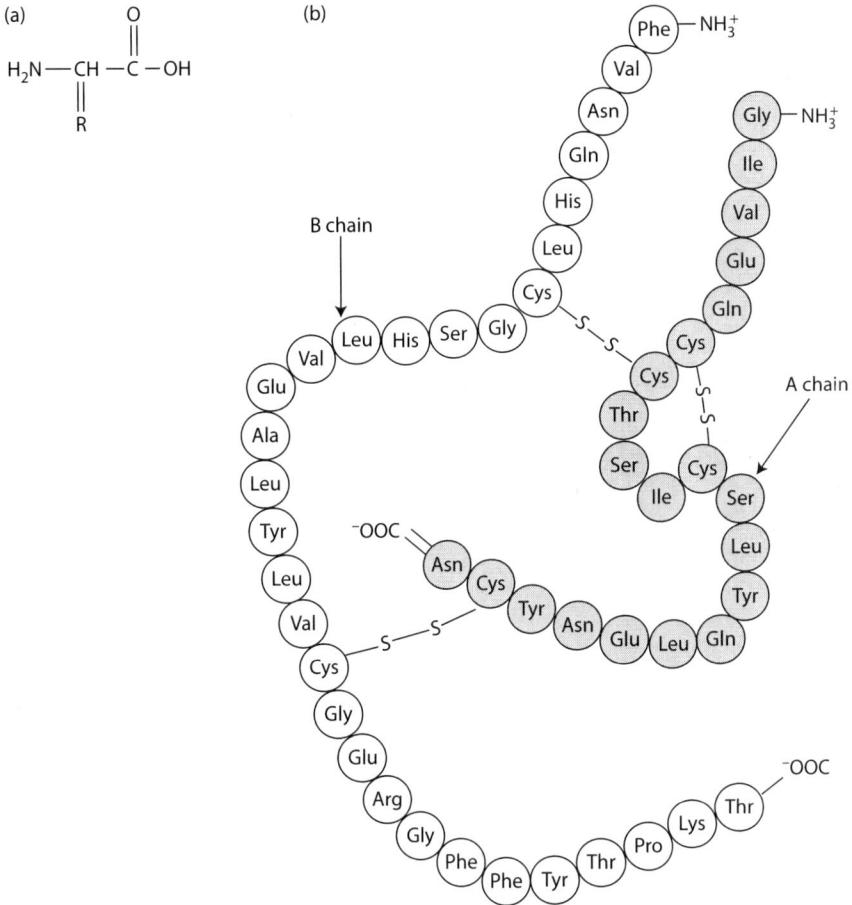

Figure 2.2 Amino acids and insulin. In (a), the basic structure of an amino acid is shown and is composed of amino (–NH₂) and carboxyl (–COOH) functional groups, with R being a side chain, which is a specific group for each amino acid. The key elements of an amino acid are hydrogen (H), nitrogen (N), carbon (C), and oxygen (O), although some amino acids contain other elements in the side chain. In (b), multiple amino acids (see Table 2.1 for the abbreviations for each amino acid) are shown that make up the protein insulin with an A chain and a B chain linked by disulfide bridges (–S–S–), making up the complete insulin molecule.

Proteins have many important functions, as listed in Table 2.2. Proteins provide structure for our tissues, organs, and bodies. For example, the structural protein collagen is the most abundant protein in mammals, making up about 25%–35% of the protein content in the whole body, and is the major protein in bone. If we were to remove the calcified material in the bones, the structure of the skeleton and even the organs would remain, because collagen is found everywhere in our bodies. Other proteins are gatekeepers of the cell and control the

Table 2.1 The 20 most common amino acids with their three-letter codes and one letter codes

Amino acid	Three-letter code	One-letter code
Alanine	ala	A
Arginine	arg	R
Asparagine	asn	N
Aspartic acid	asp	D
Cysteine	cys	C
Glutamine	gln	Q
Glutamic acid	glu	E
Glycine	gly	G
Histidine	his	H
Isoleucine	ile	I
Leucine	leu	L
Lysine	lys	K
Methionine	met	M
Phenylalanine	phe	F
Proline	pro	P
Serine	ser	S
Threonine	thr	T
Tryptophan	trp	W
Tyrosine	tyr	Y
Valine	val	V

Table 2.2 Functions of proteins

Function	Examples
Enzymes and coenzymes	RNA polymerase
Receptors	Estrogen receptor
Antibodies	Immunoglobulin G
Structural proteins	Collagen
Control membrane permeability	Calcium channel in the cell membrane
Regulate metabolites	Insulin
Bind other biomolecules as cofactors	Heme, which carries iron in hemoglobin in the blood
Control gene function	DNA polymerase (also an enzyme)
Hormones	Testosterone
Growth factors	Bone morphogenetic proteins
Cell signaling	Cyclins involved in cell growth
Contractile proteins	Actin and myosin are two proteins that make up the skeleton inside the cell (cytoskeleton)

permeability of the cell membrane, which surrounds the cytoplasm and nucleus of the cell. These proteins only allow specific molecules in and out of cells, and prevent others from entering cells. Proteins can also recognize and bind bio-molecules. These proteins can be receptors and bind biological factors such as hormones and growth factors on the cell surface. These bound receptors initiate various activities within the cells. In other words, these receptors can be likened to stockbrokers who receive our written request (hormone or growth factor) and then initiate a chain of events (cell signaling within the cell) related to our finances and thus influencing our wealth (your health). These receptors respond only to very specific factors and may be likened to your stockbroker, who only responds to your requests and not a request from your neighbor. Other proteins regulate the movement of the cytoskeleton, metabolites, and gene functions in the cell.

Another class of proteins increases the rate of chemical reactions in the body or "catalyzes" reactions. Enzymes are proteins that speed up chemical reactions. Enzymes are found mostly inside cells, often in particular types of cells and/or particular compartments of the cell, but some enzymes can be secreted outside the cell. Enzymes can be likened to high-speed internet for selling stocks in order to create the global marketplace. Amazingly, enzymes can speed the rate of a reaction by 1,000,000–1,000,000,000,000 times. Coenzymes cannot catalyze a reaction themselves, but help an enzyme to perform its function. Enzymes need to be closely regulated by cells so that a specific reaction occurs and, most importantly, ends.

POST-TRANSLATIONAL MODIFICATIONS

Interestingly, 5% of the proteome comprises enzymes that perform over 200 types of post-translational modifications. These specific enzymes are kinases, phosphatases, ligases, transferases, and proteases. Post-translational modifications are chemical modifications that change the function of proteins by regulating their activities, locations, and interactions with cellular components such as other proteins, nucleic acids, lipids, and cofactors. These post-translational modifications play a role in cancer, heart disease, diabetes, and neurodegenerative diseases, as well as normal processes in the cell, such as proliferation, cell death, and signal transduction pathways. Some of these post-translational modifications are phosphorylation, glycosylation, methylation, lipidation, ubiquitination, S-nitrosylation, and proteolysis.

With diverse types of post-translational modifications, a single protein can have multiple functions and activities based on the post-translational modifications it undergoes after it is made. This complicates the proteome of a cell (Figure 2.1) and our understanding of normal and unhealthy cell processes. Scientists seek to find specific marker proteins (biomarkers) that are unique so that they can understand specific cellular activities or so that they can target a protein as a therapy for a disease.

Post-translational modifications and their functions include:

Phosphorylation: One of the most important post-translational modifications is phosphorylation, which is a reversible process by which a phosphate group (PO_4^{-3}) is added principally to serine, threonine, or tyrosine amino acids on a protein. Phosphorylation turns many proteins on and off in numerous cellular processes, such as cell growth, death, and signaling.

Glycosylation: Protein glycosylation is one of the major post-translational modifications and has effects on protein folding, conformation, location, and stability. Thus, glycosylation can change a protein's structure and activity. Numerous types of sugar moieties are added to proteins in the process of glycosylation. Many nuclear transcription factors that regulate gene expression undergo glycosylation. Cell surface receptors and secreted proteins also undergo glycosylation prior to reaching their sites of activity.

Methylation: Methylation involves the addition of a methyl group ($-CH_3$) to nitrogen or oxygen in amino acid side chains. The enzyme methyltransferase mediates methylation, while S-adenosyl methionine (SAM) is the major methyl group donor in this very common cellular process. Methylation is a well-known mechanism of epigenetic regulation, which will be discussed in the next chapter, and influences gene expression.

Acetylation: N-acetylation occurs in 80%–90% of eukaryotic proteins, but the biological significance of this process is not completely known. An acetyl group $COCH_3$ is transferred to the nitrogen in the N-terminal amino acid methionine. The N-terminus is acetylated on growing proteins that are being translated while still attached to ribosomes. Another important acetylation occurs on the lysine of the histone N-terminus and is a method for regulating gene transcription. Histones are proteins in the nuclei that package the DNA of the chromatin, which is about 1.8 m long (about 6 feet), but when wound on the histone is about 0.09 mm, so that it can fit into the nucleus. When the histone is acetylated, it reduces the condensation or packaging of the chromosome so that transcription can take place.

Ubiquitination: Ubiquitin is a polypeptide consisting of 76 amino acids and is attached to a protein in the process called ubiquitination. This process can signal for that protein to be degraded by the proteasome, alter a protein's cellular location or activity, or promote or prevent protein interactions. A proteasome is a complex of proteins that is found inside all eukaryotic cells and in some bacteria. The proteasome degrades damaged or unneeded proteins by proteolysis.

Proteolysis: Proteolysis is a chemical reaction that breaks peptide bonds that are very stable under physiological conditions. Proteases are a family of over 11,000 enzymes that vary in their substrate specificity, mechanism of peptide cleavage, and location in the cell. Degradative proteolysis is critical for removing misfolded proteins or unassembled protein subunits in order to maintain appropriate protein concentrations within a cell. Overproduction of a particular protein can stymie normal cell activities and clog the protein-making machinery and secretion. Proteases also cleave signal peptides from proteins that are being made, as well as activating zymogens, which are inactive enzyme precursors that require cleavage in order to become active. One of the most important roles of proteases is regulating enzymatic activities in cells.

BIOMARKERS

Analysis of our proteins holds the promise that we can identify biomarkers that are unique early in the disease process. With this knowledge and the development of a therapy targeted to the biomarker, we can rid our bodies of the protein or cell with the biomarker. These biomarkers are like cruise missiles that home in on the enemy. Alternatively, biomarkers can tell us something about the cellular processes and signaling pathways that are aberrant. With this new information, we can understand the paths and processes leading to the disease, such as cancer, and find a way to stop them. The promise of proteomics is that it will provide us with biomarkers against cancer, which is the leading cause of death at approximately 7.6 million deaths worldwide per year (Ferlay et al. 2010; Jemal et al. 2011). Biomarkers are substances that are objectively measured and are determined to be indicators of a normal cellular process, pathogenic process, or a process involved in response to a pharmaceutical product.

PROTEOMICS, BIOMARKERS, AND PROSTATE CANCER

Biomarkers in personalized medicine may help to improve outcomes in male patients with prostate cancer. Prostate cancer is the second most common cancer worldwide and the sixth leading cause of death in men (Jemal et al. 2011). The current U.S. Food and Drug Administration (FDA) guidelines for prostate cancer state that detection in the blood of prostate-specific antigen (PSA), a biomarker protein produced by cells of the prostate gland, along with a digital rectal exploration for men over 50 years of age, help in diagnosing patients with prostate cancer. Unfortunately, high PSA values can also be found in patients with infection, inflammation, or benign hyperplasia (overgrowth) of the prostate, so this proteomic approach is not specific enough (Pin et al. 2013). False-positive results for cancer are sometimes found. Our doctors and their tests are not infallible, and we need to understand the disease in order to evaluate the effectiveness of therapies and so know our chances of survival or the side effects of these therapies. Figure 2.3 lists biomarkers and their advantages and disadvantages

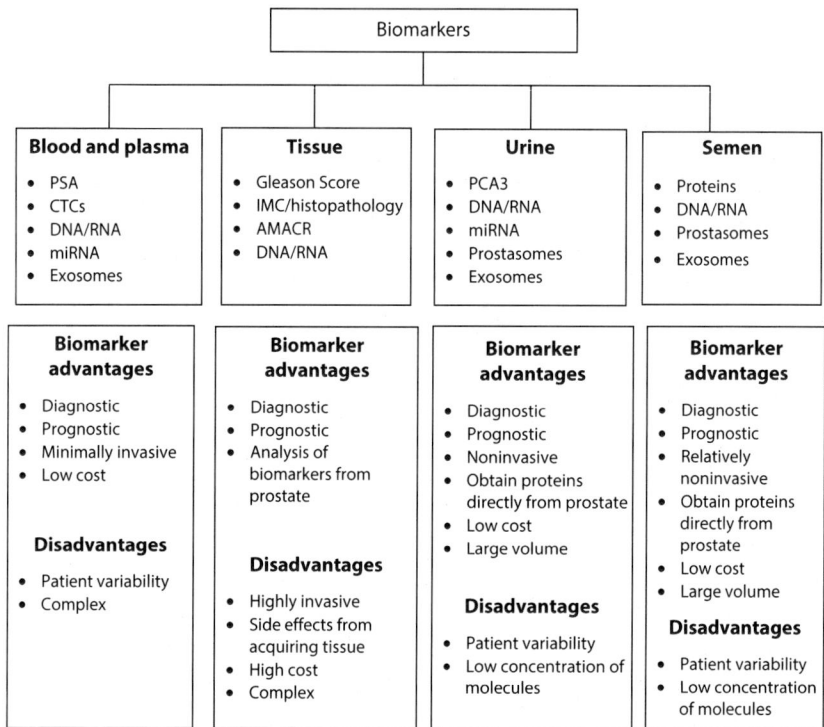

Figure 2.3 Biomarkers. This figure illustrates some of the biomarkers for prostate cancer, along with the advantages and disadvantages of biomarkers. Biomarkers are used as diagnostic and prognostic tools that are taken from blood/plasma, tissue, urine, and semen. PSA = Prostate-specific antigen, CTC = Circulating tumor cell, miRNA = MicroRNA, IMC = Immunohistochemistry, AMACR = Alpha-methylacyl-CoA racemase, PCA3 = Prostate cancer antigen 3. Patient variability can be attributed to environmental factors and the health status of the patient, such as other pre-existing diseases or conditions. (Modified from Velonas, VM, HH Woo, CG dos Remedios, and SJ Assinder. 2013. *Int J Mol Sci* 14:11034–60.)

regarding prostate cancer. Additional factors besides PSA are listed in Figure 2.3, and some discussion of them follows in this chapter.

The androgen receptor (AR) and the proteins that bind it are important in the diagnosis and treatment of prostate cancer. Androgens are male sex hormones, such as testosterone, which bind to the androgen receptor. Medical treatments for prostate cancer are based on the biology of the process by which testosterone is produced and regulated. Testosterone is the main male sex hormone, or androgen, in the blood and is able to fuel prostate cancer. Approximately 85%–90% of testosterone is produced in the testicles and 10% in the adrenal glands. The pathway by which testosterone is regulated is as follows: the hypothalamus in the brain detects low testosterone levels and releases luteinizing hormone-releasing hormone (LHRH; also called gonadotropin-releasing hormone), which travels to the pituitary gland, where it binds LHRH receptors. The pituitary responds by releasing a hormone called luteinizing hormone (LH), which travels to receptors in the testicles and stimulates the production of testosterone. Testosterone levels increase and are then detected by the hypothalamus, which then stops the production of LHRH until testosterone levels are low and the cycle begins again. Nature has created checks and balances for regulating testosterone levels. Testosterone and dihydrotestosterone need to bind the AR and activate it so that it can regulate gene expression. Some of the genes that are activated through the AR are important for the development and maintenance of male sexual characteristics (Mooradian et al. 1987).

The personalized medicine approaches to prostate cancer are based on proteomics (proteins such as hormones and their receptors) and target different steps discussed in the biological pathway outlined above. Different drugs were created in order to inhibit different steps in the production and action of testosterone on prostate cancer cells and thus limit tumor growth: LHRH agonists, LHRH antagonists, antiandrogens, and testosterone synthesis inhibitors. Agonists are chemicals that bind to a receptor and activate the biological response associated with the receptor. An antagonist is a protein that blocks the action of an agonist. The goal of this therapy is to inhibit the production of testosterone, which increases prostate cancer.

Drugs that stop the production and action of testosterone include LHRH agonists, LHRH antagonists, antiandrogens, and testosterone synthesis inhibitors:

1. LHRH agonists suppress the pituitary's response to testosterone. LHRH agonists are chemicals that mimic naturally occurring LHRH without being identical to it. They are able to bind to the LHRH receptor and stay bound. As a result of the prolonged presence of the LHRH agonists and persistent release of LH, there is a sudden rise in testosterone. This spike in testosterone level is known as a "hormone flare," which can feel uncomfortable in men, just like "hot flashes" in women. After several days, the LHRH receptors become desensitized due to constant binding and the receptors are downregulated. LH production decreases and testosterone levels drop.

2. LHRH antagonists stop the production of testosterone in the testes and adrenal glands. LHRH antagonists are small molecules that bind to the LHRH receptors but do not activate the receptors; instead, they block its activation and no LH is produced. The testicles stop producing testosterone.

3. Antiandrogens inhibit the action of testosterone. When antiandrogens bind to ARs within the prostate cancer cells, testosterone is unable to bind to its receptors and is unable to stimulate cell growth to the same extent. This slows down the growth of prostate cancer.

4. Testosterone synthesis inhibitors: The FDA has recently approved androgen synthesis inhibitors in order to stop testosterone production from cells. This new treatment is especially important for men who have "castration-resistant prostate cancer." This type of prostate cancer can grow even when the testicles no longer supply hormone, because some cancers continue to thrive on very low levels of testosterone that remain or are still produced in the patient. Other names for this "castration-resistant" cancer include androgen-independent, androgen-resistant, or androgen-insensitive cancer.

As in breast cancer, a biopsy of the prostate is used to determine the stage of the disease by microscopic analysis of a small piece of the prostate. The Gleason Grading System (ranging from 2 to 10) is the method by which the pathologist assesses the tissue in order to help evaluate the prognosis of men with prostate cancer (Epstein 2010). The identification of the glands and the pattern of the cells in the prostate tissue are some of the features that pathologists use to determine the Gleason score (Figure 2.3). With a piece of prostate tissue from the biopsy, immunohistochemistry (IHC) can be performed in order to determine the proteins expressed in the prostate gland. IHC is a technique by which antigens/proteins in cells of the tissue are detected by binding antibodies that are specific to them. The antigen–antibody complex is visualized by different methods using an enzyme, such as peroxidase, which catalyzes a color-producing reaction in the tissue. Alternatively, the antibody can be tagged with a fluorophore (fluorescent marker) such as fluorescein or rhodamine in a process called immunofluorescence in order to identify specific cells with that marker.

Besides the Gleason Grading System, the age of the patient is important in determining treatment. With elderly men above the age of 70 with a low Gleason score, the approach is to carefully monitor the patient, but not to operate. The reason behind not operating is due to the slow growth rate of the cancer. There may be complications from surgery such as incontinence and impotence, which can dramatically affect a person's lifestyle and their well-being. However, 75% of the prostate cancer cases treated by surgery and/or pharmacologic castration result in tumor regression (Pin et al. 2013). Here is an example in which both proteomics and the personal information of the patient are combined in order to determine what the best therapy is for the patient.

With surgery and pharmacologic castration (blocking testosterone production or the AR), there are a number of problems that can occur, such as the development of androgen-independent cancer cells that grow and metastasize to another tissue and create more tumors. This phenomenon complicates the treatment of these patients, since therapies targeting the AR would be ineffective in stopping the disease. We do not know why this can happen, or which patients are at risk. We do know that during prostate cancer progression, many changes in proteins and their pathways arise, especially due to the accumulation of gene mutations or modifications to gene expression. DNA–RNA can be used as a biomarker (Figure 2.3). So far, more than 605 mutations have been found for the AR gene that can modify its expression and signaling pathways (Gottlieb et al. 2004). This is one of the pitfalls of proteomics and genomics, in that changes in proteins and genes in cancer can complicate the process for designing a pharmaceutical therapy to target the disease. Another issue in many cancers, including prostate cancer, is that the cells in the tissue or stroma around the tumor secrete growth factors that promote the progression of the tumor (Feldman et al. 2001), and this can also influence cancer outcomes. How should we target the stroma therapeutically?

The analysis of proteins, their functions, and signaling pathways is being undertaken in order to determine why androgen-independent cancer cells develop and to find a more definitive marker or biomarkers that can distinguish aggressive prostate cancers from less aggressive ones, and with this knowledge, tailor the therapy for that particular patient. Of interest is that obese patients have a higher risk of developing prostate cancer and that the fat around the prostate can participate in the cancer process and progression (Payton 2012). Obesity also increases the risk for breast cancer and causes less effective responses to drugs that would inhibit recurrence (Azrad and Demark-Wahnefried 2014). Therefore, if we want to rid ourselves of cancer and take advantage of the new therapeutics coming from proteomics, we must also play our part and lose weight appropriately (not too fast or in an unhealthy manner) so that our responses to the drugs given to us by our doctors is effective and the chance of cancer recurrence is lessened.

Biomarkers also have value for understanding the disease process at the cellular and tissue levels, so that metabolites of the early disease process can be identified and the diseases eradicated before they involve major organs. Cancer cells, such as in prostate cancer, are known to release exosomes, which are 30–100-nm diameter mini-cell-like vacuoles that are involved in cell-to-cell communication. They have the characteristic surface proteins of their cell of origin and some specific intracellular proteins within the vacuole. Exosomes probably play a role in tumorigenesis and are being studied by scientists as a possible diagnostic tool (Velonas et al. 2013).

Additional materials from cells that could perhaps serve as biomarkers are prostasomes, which are from healthy and malignant prostate acini cells and have a size of 4–500 nm. Prostasomes are involved in the liquefaction of semen and enhancement of sperm motility. Prostasomes also have immunosuppressive, antioxidant, and antibacterial properties. In addition, there can be circulating cancer cells in the blood in some patients that can be assayed for disease prognosis. Other biomarkers that are being developed for prostate cancer are alpha-methylacyl-CoA racemase (AMACR), which is expressed within prostate adenocarcinoma cells, and prostate cancer antigen 3 (PCA3). PCA3 is a gene that is found in a noncoding RNA that is expressed in the human prostate and is overexpressed in prostate cancer (Figure 2.3).

A pitfall in the proteomic approach is that the proteins at the tissue level may not reflect the proteins in the circulation, such that we must examine both sources for biomarkers. Thus, multiple assays and multiple biomarkers need to be examined in order to make a diagnosis of prostate cancer, patient prognosis, and therapy. Tumor tissue is composed of many different subpopulations of different types of cells that talk to each other through biochemical signals that promote and sustain tumor growth. This makes it difficult to know which type of cell to target in order to halt cancer progression. Some of these issues can be solved to a certain extent by new techniques, such as cell sorting of the tumor cells in order to determine cell differences and laser capture microdissection of individual cells. Both of these techniques allow scientists to subculture these cells outside of the body in order to learn more about their protein markers and activities. Proteins can also be extracted from specific cells by specific techniques such as microarrays and mass spectrometry. Since tumors are heterogeneous, even in one person, probably the most accurate screening tests in the future will involve a multiplex panel of biomarkers, and their success will be determined by technologies such as bioinformatics, which involve large-scale patient screening for biomarkers in a clinical setting. Without bioinformatics, which encompasses software tools in order to store, retrieve, organize, and analyze this biological information that identifies key players in a disease, we would not be able to use successfully the information gained in the laboratory for personalized medicine. However, all of these tests can be very expensive to undergo and for our medical system to absorb.

As can be seen from our previous discussion of prostate cancer, proteomics seeks to find: (1) a protein or several proteins that can be used to detect cancer in an individual—this biomarker(s) needs to be highly sensitive and specific for the cancer; (2) the proteomic approach, which tries to identify proteins that predict whether this cancer is very aggressive and also if it is likely to recur; and (3) another goal of proteomics is to find proteins that predict a patient's response to a particular treatment so that the most appropriate therapy can be chosen. Most important would be to find biomarkers in the blood or other biological fluids, such as blood/plasma, urine, or semen (Figure 2.3), which can easily identify those patients who are at risk of a particular type of cancer, such as prostate cancer, or have an early form of the disease.

METABOLOMICS

Another relatively new field of research for identifying metabolites of disease is called metabolomics. Metabolomics is the study of chemical processes involving metabolites. These metabolites are similar to fingerprints that, when recognized, tell you who is the culprit causing these changes in the body. The metabolome is the collection of metabolites in a specific tissue or cell that describe in more detail the cellular process(es) of interest. For example, ancient cultures placed ants near a urine sample of a patient. If that patient had diabetes with high levels of glucose/sugar, then the ants would be drawn to the urine. We are more sophisticated now, as various proteins and enzymes can be identified in human fluids—sweat, urine, saliva, and blood—that can provide information on physiology, cellular processes, and ultimately health (Figure 2.3).

The history of metabolomics is recent, with Dr. Marjorie Horning in 1971 demonstrating that a technique called gas chromatography (GC)–mass spectroscopy could be used to measure metabolites in human urine and tissue extracts (Horning et al. 1975). The GC–mass spectroscopy instrument uses the GC portion to separate chemical mixtures into pure chemicals based on their ability to evaporate into a gas. It is similar to a race in which runners reach the finish line based on how fast they are running compared to everyone else. By the time they reach the finish line, each runner has separated themselves from the crowd at the starting line. In general, small molecules will travel more quickly than larger molecules. Then, the mass spectrometer identifies and quantifies the chemicals. This is accomplished by breaking apart each molecule that travels through GC with a stream of electrons. The molecules are broken up into ions that then pass through an electromagnetic field that allows the ions to travel differentially through a filter that scans them for their particular mass. A detector counts the number of ions with a specific mass and a computer determines the mass spectrum. The particular pattern in the spectrum can be used to identify the chemical.

Another technique—nuclear magnetic resonance (NMR) spectroscopy—uses the magnetic properties of atomic nuclei to give the structure, reaction state, and chemical environment of molecules, which are unique for each molecule. NMR is then able to identify the molecule. In 1974, Seely et al. used NMR to demonstrate that 90% of the adenosine triphosphate (ATP) in muscle is complexed with magnesium (Hoult et al. 1974). In 1984, Nicholson et al. showed that NMR could diagnose diabetes mellitus (Bales et al. 1984; Nicholson et al. 1984). In 2007, Dr. David Wishart from the University of Alberta, Canada, and head of the Human Metabolome Project, completed the first draft of the human metabolome, consisting of approximately 2500 metabolites, 1200 drugs, and 3500 food components (Wishart 2007), which is still being completed for the diagnosis of biological processes and their diseases.

PROTEOMICS, BIOMARKERS, AND BREAST CANCER

Breast cancer accounts for 14% of cancer-related deaths. Breast cancer has increased over the past decade and is expected to continue increasing. The problem with breast cancer is that the tumors in each person differ greatly (i.e., they are heterogeneous) in their protein and gene expression, just as we are all different in appearance from each other, yet we have some similar structures, such as noses, eyes, and legs. This heterogeneity is a particular problem for breast cancer metastasis, in which a cell or cells from the primary tumor have the ability to migrate through the surrounding tissue, enter the circulation, and travel to another tissue site, where they create secondary tumors. The pitfall in proteomics for breast cancer is that these metastatic breast cancer cells in their new tissue sites frequently have different properties, such as different receptors or other cell surface proteins, and no longer respond to the targeted therapy to that receptor or surface protein of the primary tumor. These metastases are the causes of the great majority of deaths from breast cancer.

Another pitfall is that some tumors can develop resistance to previous chemotherapy treatments. Therefore, early detection of breast cancer is very important for survival. I was lucky, since my breast cancer was found early on a routine mammogram. Thus, a therapy based on results from proteomics can be developed from the primary tumor, but it may or may not work for metastatic tumors. The issue of tumor heterogeneity is also found with other cancers, such as melanoma, a cancer of the skin. This tumor heterogeneity is one of the reasons why skin cancer is dangerous, and its early detection is important for survival. Melanoma originates from DNA damage due to ultraviolet (UV) radiation from the sun.

Breast carcinoma is the type of breast cancer that is most commonly found in patients, and carcinoma refers to a cancer that begins in a tissue that lines the inner and outer body surfaces: epithelial cells. These cells become transformed and behave abnormally or exhibit malignant properties and become cancerous. Four major subtypes, reflecting different gene expression and proteins in different cells, have been found in breast cancer tissue, which is one of the reasons for the disease's heterogeneity. A short description of these subtypes is important for understanding the disease and the targeted proteomic-based therapies. These tissue subtypes express different proteins, which are the bases for some of the medical treatments in personalized medicine.

We will briefly discuss these breast cancer subtypes and the treatments that have been developed in order to target the cancer in personalized medicine (Figure 2.4). These subtypes are identified by taking a biopsy of the breast tissue and using IHC to determine tissue appearance and protein/gene expression so as to delineate the type of breast cancer: luminal (subtypes a and b), human epidermal growth factor-2 (HER-2)-enriched, basal-like, and normal breast-like subtypes (Perou et al. 2000; Sorlie et al. 2003; Lam et al. 2014). Of course, the normal breast-like subtype is normal breast tissue, but islands of cancer cells can also be found intermixed with normal breast tissue. The luminal a subtype

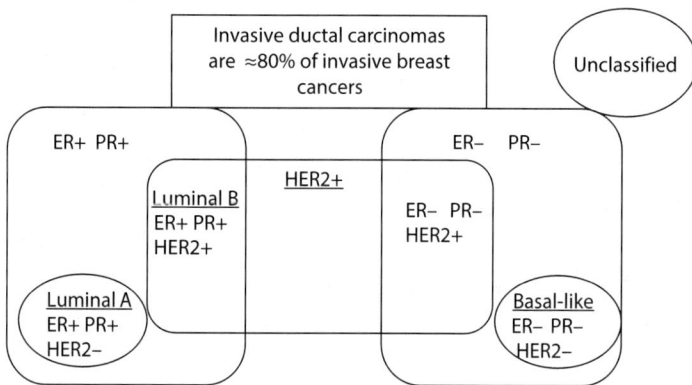

Figure 2.4 Breast cancer subtypes. Invasive ductal carcinomas comprise approximately 80% of breast cancers and consist of different subtypes depending on their protein/gene expression of particular proteins and hormone receptors. These subtypes are luminal a, luminal b, human epidermal growth factor-2 (HER-2) enriched, and basal-like. These subtypes can express different hormone receptors, such as the estrogen receptor, progesterone receptor, or HER-2. Breast cancer subtypes can be either positive (+) or negative (–) for these receptors. (Modified from Sandhu, R, JS Parker, WD Jones, CA Livasy, and WB Coleman. 2010. *Lab Med* 41(6):364–72.)

represents about 50% of breast carcinomas, and "luminal" refers to the proteins expressed in the opening (lumen) of the mammary ducts in the breast. The luminal a subtype of cells also expresses specific proteins, such as the estrogen and progesterone hormone receptors and epithelial protein markers cytokeratin 8 and 18. They undergo slower cell growth than other cancers. The luminal b subtype has some of the same markers, but has a different tissue appearance, which shows increased disease progression compared to the luminal a subtype. Most medical treatments for breast cancer involve surgery, often chemotherapy and radiation. However, those tumors that are estrogen receptor positive depend on estrogen for their growth, so they can be treated with drugs to reduce either the effect of estrogen (e.g., tamoxifen) or the level of estrogen (e.g., aromatase inhibitors). Recent literature suggests that taking aromatase inhibitors for 5 years may improve cancer-free survival compared to tamoxifen, but any difference in survival benefit from either drug is still controversial (Van Asten et al. 2014).

Approximately 4%–7% of breast carcinomas are classified HER-2 enriched, in that they overexpress epidermal growth factor (EGF) receptors in the cell membrane, which accelerate cell growth. Why is this important? If we personalize the analysis of the cancer and determine that it is HER-2 positive, then these patients are given targeted treatments with a monoclonal antibody, which binds specifically to the HER-2 receptor, interferes with its function, and prevents additional cancer growth. Monoclonal antibodies are created by stimulating identical immune cells to bind to only one specific protein sequence—in this case the HER-2 receptor—and produce a monoclonal antibody to it. This monoclonal antibody has been marketed as trastuzumab with drug names of Herclon and Herceptin, and in combination with other chemotherapies, has improved the outcomes and survival of these breast cancer patients.

The basal-like subtype of breast cancer tissue comprises about 10%–20% of breast carcinomas and is characterized by the overexpression of genes and proteins related to the basal layer of the mammary duct. The basal layer refers to the "myoepithelial" layer that is on the opposite side of the luminal side and is the innermost layer of the cells in the mammary duct. It has its own specific protein markers, but it is also negative for the three protein markers found in the other types of breast cancer discussed above: estrogen receptor, progesterone receptor, and HER-2. This type of cancer is often called triple-negative breast cancer, and usually has a higher histologic grade with a faster rate of cell growth. At the time of my writing, 11 proteins have been identified that are able to determine disease outcome in 89% of triple-negative breast cancer patients (Lam et al. 2014). Perhaps by the time that this book is published, a personalized therapy for this type of breast cancer will have been developed.

PROTEOMICS AND ATHEROSCLEROSIS

The proteomic scientific approach is not only used to find cures for cancer, but also for the treatment of other diseases. One example is vascular proteomics, which encompasses heart attacks (myocardial infarction), stroke (cerebral ischemia), and gangrene. These diseases are due to blood vessel dysfunction and plaque formation. Plaque formation is not felt by the patient or found by a physician until plaques reach a critical size and change, leading to atherosclerosis. Atherosclerosis is the process of chronic inflammation with the development of plaques. Plaques are composed of lipids, different types of cells (such as white blood cells), calcification, and fibrous elements in the medium and large arteries (the vessels that move the blood away from the heart to the tissues, and most often contain oxygenated blood). These plaques cause the arteries to harden and lose their elasticity, making it difficult for the blood to flow through the body and nourish tissues. Other related terms that are used are arteriosclerosis, which is a general term describing any hardening and loss of elasticity of medium or large arteries, and arteriolosclerosis, which is any hardening and loss of elasticity of arterioles (small arteries). Therefore, finding novel biomarkers early in the disease process is critical for early medical intervention.

A perfect biomarker for atherosclerosis has not yet been discovered (Barderas et al. 2013). Some promising biomarker candidates have been identified, such as C-reactive protein (CRP), which is found in the blood and synthesized by the liver in response to inflammation. CRP binds phosphocholine expressed on the surfaces of dead and dying cells, which activates the immune system. However, when assayed in patients, it only slightly improves the clinical prognostic model for cardiovascular diseases that included age, sex, smoking status, blood pressure, history of diabetes, and total cholesterol level (Emerging Risk Factors Collaboration 2012). Again, personal information is critical for our doctors to determine what the best therapy is for us, and so we must be truthful when discussing our habits and personal history. Other inflammatory markers have been studied, such as CD40L, monocyte attractant protein-1 (MCP-1), adhesion molecules, myeloperoxidase, and several cytokines, but none have demonstrated consistent predictive value in the clinic (Barderas et al. 2013). There are many potential markers for prostate cancer that scientists have found, but a new therapeutic approach has yet to be developed (Pin et al. 2013).

One of the pitfalls in proteomics is finding the correct biomarker for the disease. The diversity of the cells and metabolites in the disease process makes it difficult to locate the correct biomarker. Vascular cells differ depending upon in which blood vessel they are located, and a host of different immune cells are involved at different stages of the disease. Metabolites are small molecules that participate in chemical processes occurring in the body and are necessary for the maintenance, growth, and normal functioning of cells. These metabolites differ depending on the stage of the disease and can be found in tissue, urine, blood plasma, and serum. So where and how do you find the correct and best biomarker in order to predict cardiovascular disease progression?

The promise of proteomics is the "omics," which is the technology that is being developed in order to gain knowledge of the whole system, including different stages, cells, and metabolites. Mega-computers are needed in order to hold proteomic information, sort it, and develop an understanding of the disease process and prognosis for a particular patient. Many other diseases, including atherosclerosis and cancer, are complex, multifactorial diseases, requiring a more global biological analysis or systems biology approach in order to assay multiple proteins in various networks at different times and so determine potential biomarkers. With the use of bioinformatics to identify key players in a disease, the hope is to find a panel of biomarkers that will predict disease progression and individual patient prognoses. However, there is a pitfall in relying only on computer-generated information, since it is the human being, such as a doctor, who has the ultimate responsibility for any prognosis and treatment. In Chapter 11 on ethics, a discussion of this topic is presented. Ultimately, a doctor should be the one to make sense of and check any treatment regimens generated by bioinformatics programs for personalized medicine. Our doctors who treat us are only as good as our knowledge of the specific disease process and treatment tools we develop.

REFERENCES

Azrad, M and W Demark-Wahnefried. 2014. The association between adiposity and breast cancer recurrence and survival: A review of the recent literature. *Curr Nutr Rep* 3(1):9–15.

Bales, JR, DP Higham, I Howe, JK Nicholson, and PJ Sadler. 1984. Use of high-resolution proton nuclear magnetic resonance spectroscopy for rapid multi-component analysis of urine. *Clin Chem* 30(3):426–32.

Barderas, MG, F Vivanco, and G Alvarez-Llamas. 2013. Vascular proteomics. *Methods Mol Biol* 1000:1–20.

Emerging Risk Factors Collaboration. 2012. C-reactive protein, fibrinogen, and cardiovascular disease prediction. *N Engl J Med* 367(14):1310–20.

Epstein, JI. 2010. An update of the Gleason grading system. *J Urol* 183(2):433–40.

Feldman, KS, K Sahasrabudhe, MD Lawlor, SL Wilson, CH Lang, and WJ Scheuchenzuber. 2001. *In vitro* and *in vivo* inhibition of LPS-stimulated tumor necrosis factor-alpha secretion by the gallotannin beta-D-pentagalloylglucose. *Bioorg Med Chem Lett* 11(14):1813–5.

Ferlay, J, DM Parkin, and E Steliarova-Foucher. 2010. Estimates of cancer incidence and mortality in Europe in 2008. *Eur J Cancer* 46(4):765–81.

Gottlieb, B, LK Beitel, JH Wu, and M Trifiro. 2004. The androgen receptor gene mutations database (ARDB): 2004 update. *Hum Mutat* 23(6):527–33.

Horning, MG, J Nowlin, M Stafford, K Lertratanangkoon, KR Sommer, RM Hill, and RN Stillwell. 1975. The use of gas chromatographic–mass spectrometric–computer systems in pharmacokinetic studies. *J Chromatogr* 112:605–15.

Hoult, DI, SJ Busby, DG Gadian, GK Radda, RE Richards, and PJ Seeley. 1974. Observation of tissue metabolites using 31P nuclear magnetic resonance. *Nature* 252 (5481):285–7.

Jemal, A, F Bray, MM Center, J Ferlay, E Ward, and D Forman. 2011. Global cancer statistics. *CA Cancer J Clin* 61(2):69–90.

Jensen, ON. 2004. Modification-specific proteomics: Characterization of post-translational modifications by mass spectrometry. *Curr Opin Chem Biol* 8:33–41.

Lam, SW, SM de Groot, AH Honkoop et al., and Group Dutch Breast Cancer Research. 2014. Paclitaxel and bevacizumab with or without capecitabine as first-line treatment for HER2-negative locally recurrent or metastatic breast cancer: A multicentre, open-label, randomised phase 2 trial. *Eur J Cancer* 50(18):3077–3088.

Mooradian, AD, JE Morley, and SG Korenman. 1987. Biological actions of androgens. *Endocr Rev* 8(1):1–28.

Nicholson, JK, MP O'Flynn, PJ Sadler, AF Macleod, SM Juul, and PH Sonksen. 1984. Proton-nuclear-magnetic-resonance studies of serum, plasma and urine from fasting normal and diabetic subjects. *Biochem J* 217(2):365–75.

Payton, S. 2012. Prostate cancer: Periprostatic fat is a risk factor for prostate cancer detection. *Nat Rev Urol* 9(4):180.

Perou, CM, T Sorlie, MB Eisen et al. 2000. Molecular portraits of human breast tumours. *Nature* 406(6797):747–52.

Pin, E, C Fredolini, and EF Petricoin 3rd. 2013. The role of proteomics in prostate cancer research: Biomarker discovery and validation. *Clin Biochem* 46(6):524–38.

Sandhu, R, JS Parker, WD Jones, CA Livasy, and WB Coleman. 2010. Microarray-based gene expression profiling for molecular classification of breast cancer and identification of new targets for therapy. *Lab Med* 41(6):364–72.

Sorlie, T, R Tibshirani, J Parker et al. 2003. Repeated observation of breast tumor subtypes in independent gene expression data sets. *Proc Natl Acad Sci USA* 100(14):8418–23.

Van Asten, K, P Neven, A Lintermans, H Wildiers, and R Paridaens. 2014. Aromatase inhibitors in the breast cancer clinic: Focus on exemestane. *Endocr Relat Cancer* 21(1):R31–49.

Velonas, VM, HH Woo, CG dos Remedios, and SJ Assinder. 2013. Current status of biomarkers for prostate cancer. *Int J Mol Sci* 14:11034–60.

Wishart, DS. 2007. Human Metabolome Database: Completing the "human parts list." *Pharmacogenomics* 8(7):683–6.

3

Epigenetics

Would you want to sequence your own genome and find out what genes you have?

Today, sequencing of your personal genome is possible. If it is cost that is a problem, then realize that the sequencing of the first human genome required about $2.7 million, and now the cost has dropped to approximately $1500/person. Sequencing of a genome can take as little as 50 hours to accomplish. By sequencing your genome, you would know if you have any mutations or a gene that could predispose you to a particular disease. However, even with a mutation or toxic gene, you may not express the disease. Twin studies have found that both twins can have the gene for a disease and only one may develop that disease in their lifetime (Weksberg et al. 2002; Fraga et al. 2005). Would you want to know about your genes no matter what happens in your lifetime, or would this information weigh too heavily on you and cause undue stress and worry? Alternatively, would this information encourage you to take better care of yourself and cause you to try and offset expressing a disease? Another item for thought is: how would you protect this information so that no one discriminates against you in any way? Science is never as simple as reading your DNA sequence and predicting the future. No one—not even your doctor—can be a fortune-teller.

The DNA profile of your genes is further complicated by epigenetics, which are inherited changes in DNA expression that occur in the absence of changes in the primary DNA sequence. So, knowing all of the genes and even proteins in the body does not necessarily determine whether a mutation or particular gene will ever be expressed. A person may have a deleterious gene, but due to epigenetics, it may be diminished in expression or not expressed. Important epigenetic processes, such as DNA methylation, histone acetylation, and deacetylation, and the effects of noncoding RNAs have been recognized in diseases such as cancer, inflammation, diabetes, and central nervous system disorders.

Many of these epigenetic events lead to gene silencing that is inherited from one generation to the next. Genes can be turned off by RNA when antisense transcripts of RNA, such as noncoding RNA or RNA interference (RNAi), are formed and typically cause the destruction of specific mRNAs by triggering histone modifications or DNA methylation (Figure 3.1). Many small RNAs affect

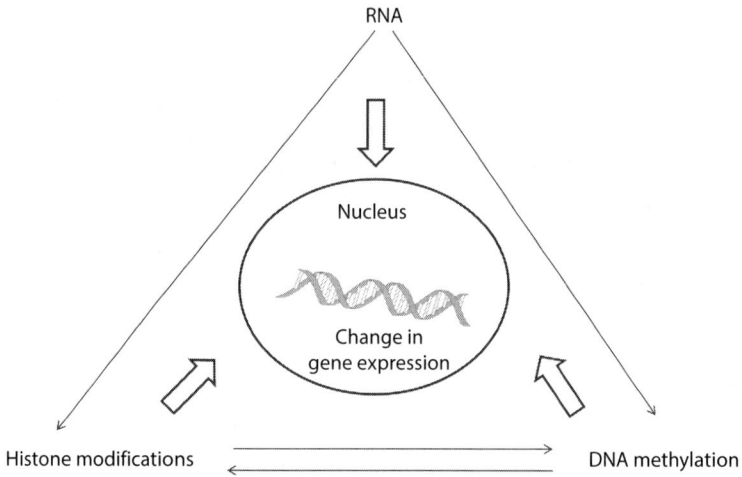

Figure 3.1 Epigenetics. Interactions between RNA, histones, and DNA methylation cause heritable changes in gene expression. The RNAs such as microRNAs (miRNAs), RNA interference (RNAi), and noncoding RNAs can modify gene activities. Histone modifications involving acetylation and deacetylation or methylation can also change the activities of genes in the chromatin. For example, deacetylation of histones will cause the chromatin to condense, forming heterochromatin, which is inactive, while acetylation reverses this process and activates the gene. DNA methylation causes a change in the structure of DNA, thus modifying a gene's interaction with the nuclear machinery needed for transcription, which alters the gene's expression.

gene expression and control, and they are generally inhibitory. Therefore, these RNAs and the processes that regulate their mechanisms of action are referred to as RNA silencing and their main categories are small interfering RNAs or RNA silencing (siRNAs), microRNAs (miRNAs), and Piwi-interacting RNAs (piRNAs). These epigenetic processes will be discussed in light of particular diseases.

DIABETES AND EPIGENETICS

Diabetes mellitus, which we refer to as diabetes, is a disease of glucose homeostasis that affects more than 24 million Americans and 382 million individuals in the world (Guariguata et al. 2014). There are two types of diabetes; type 1 and type 2. Type 1 diabetes is due to autoimmune destruction of a particular cell in the pancreas, the β-cell, which regulates sugar/glucose metabolism and synthesizes insulin (Figure 3.2). Researchers are still trying to get a clear picture of what causes diabetes—they have found that genes do not tell the whole story, and that environmental factors also play a role. Research has shown that only 15% of people with type 1 diabetes have an affected first-degree relative; therefore, type 1 diabetes is not necessarily hereditary.

In autoimmunity, immune cells attack healthy cells in the body and cause an autoimmune disease. Each person's immune system protects them from disease

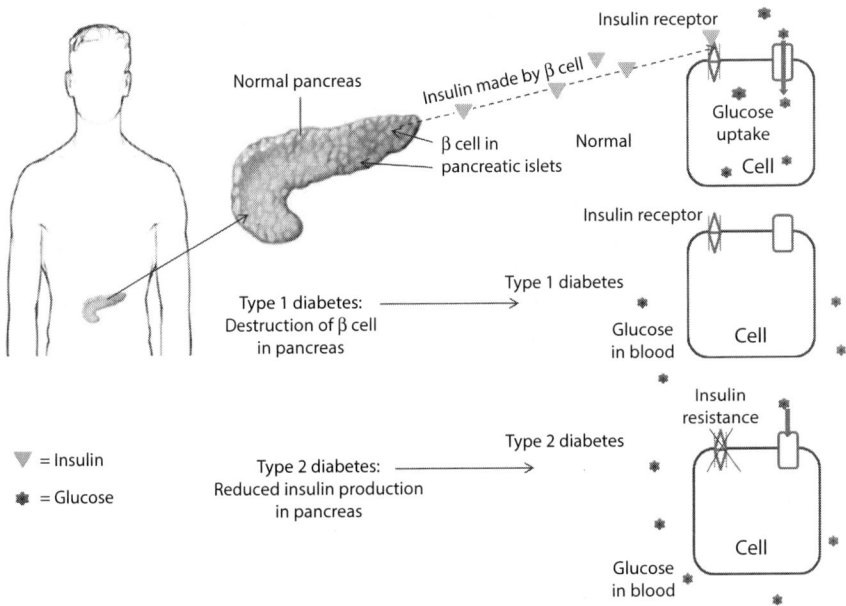

Figure 3.2 Diabetes. The pancreas maintains normal glucose levels by producing insulin in its β-cells. The insulin binds to its receptors on cells in the body and promotes glucose uptake from the blood into cells. Glucose is needed for metabolism in cells and tissues. In type 1 diabetes, the β-cells are unable to produce insulin in order to handle the glucose in the bloodstream, and eventually the β-cells are destroyed. Glucose cannot be taken into cells and their levels become high in the blood. Type 2 diabetes is more prevalent and some insulin is produced, but the cells do not respond to insulin properly, so glucose levels rise in the blood. As the disease progresses, a lack of insulin may develop.

and infections by recognizing pathogens, such as viruses and parasites, as different from your healthy tissue. The reason or reasons for autoimmunity arise from interactions between the environment and genetic and epigenetic factors that result in changes in the complex network of interactions between immune cells and the cells of the body. There are more than 80 types of immune diseases and they affect over 50 million Americans according to the American Autoimmune Related Diseases Association (AARDA), while the National Institute of Health in Washington, D.C., only recognizes half of that number due to differences in evaluating these diseases.

The more common type of diabetes—type 2—is due to insulin resistance, dysregulation of liver sugar metabolism (gluconeogenesis), and progressive β-cell dysfunction (Figure 3.2). Type 2 diabetes often starts in adulthood, while type 1 diabetes develops in children or young adults. Both types of diabetes have a familial predisposition (i.e., genetic susceptibility). Genome-wide association study (GWAS) point to the presence of gene polymorphisms (genes that express different physical characteristics in an organism) that contribute to β-cell failure and the development of diabetes. For type 1 diabetes, GWAS have identified genes that regulate autoimmunity and thus the immune system in the body. However, some of these same genes that are important in immunity have also been found in the β-cells of the pancreas. For type 2 diabetes, GWAS implicate genes that predispose individuals to β-cell malfunction when insulin is unregulated (Johnson and Evans-Molina 2015). Therefore, for both types of diabetes, the β-cells of the pancreas are affected. Not only are the genes that are implicated in diabetes found among family members, but epigenetics also appears to play an important role in these families.

DIABETES AND DNA METHYLATION

DNA methylation is a molecular phenomenon of epigenetics in which a methyl group ($-CH_3$) is added to a cytosine (C) that is next to a guanine (G) in the DNA sequence, creating what is called CpG. Methylation is like a light switch that can turn on and off a gene's expression. Approximately 70% of these CpG sites are hypermethylated in the mammalian genome, which causes these genes to be suppressed (i.e., dimming or turning off the light). The remaining unmethylated sites are often found in promoter regions of genes, the DNA regions that initiate transcription and activate gene expression, turning on the light. Methylation of DNA is important in cell differentiation when inappropriate genes are suppressed in particular cells, such that they only express genes for that cell and tissue. You would not want your bone cells to produce insulin, or your pancreatic cells to produce bone matrix. Methylation varies from cell type to cell type in order to create specific gene expression profiles depending on the tissue.

An example of epigenetics related to methylation and unmethylation is found on chromosome 6q24, where unmethylation causes a rare form of transient neonatal diabetes (TND). A few days after birth, TND results in β-cell dysfunction, which resolves in infancy, but predisposes that person to diabetes as they age (Temple and Shield 2010). Analysis of cadavers has also shown altered patterns of methylation, mostly hypermethylation, in 254 genes of islets in the pancreases of those who were diabetic in life compared to those people who were not diabetic (Volkmar et al. 2012). One gene that affects cell survival in pancreatic islets from people with type 2 diabetes is the CD5R1 gene. This gene encodes a cyclin-dependent kinase 5 (CDK5) regulatory subunit protein that is often found to be hypomethylated (i.e., active) in the pancreas of type 2 diabetes patients (Wei et al. 2005). CDK5 is activated in the β-cells by high glucose levels and proinflammatory cytokines, and results in decreased transcription of the insulin gene (i.e., decreasing insulin levels) and pancreatic and duodenal homeobox-1 (Pdx-1), which play important roles in β-cell development.

Another interesting example of epigenetic methylation comes from the study of mothers who were obese and then underwent weight reduction after gastric bypass surgery. Children who were born before or after the procedure had different DNA methylation patterns in the genes involved in glucose regulation and inflammation, even though they were siblings (Guénard et al. 2013; Patti 2013). Those children born after gastric bypass surgery were less obese and had improved cardiometabolic risk profiles compared to their siblings born before their mothers had surgery. Again, we see that obesity is detrimental to a mother's health and can affect her children for their whole life. This hypomethylation results in an inability to properly regulate glucose metabolism. Thus, epigenetics has far-reaching effects on the health status of families, and complicates our ability to predict gene function from the DNA sequence of an individual.

HISTONES AND EPIGENETICS

Histone modifications are also part of epigenetics (Figure 3.1). Histones are proteins that package the DNA on chromosomes in the nucleus of the cell and affect gene expression. During the development of an organism, the N-terminal tails of the histones can be modified through acetylation, methylation, ubiquitination, and phosphorylation in order to differentially activate different genes, like a light switch (Johnson and Evans-Molina 2015). These patterns can be passed from parents to their children.

Continuing with the example of diabetes, these different histone modifications are differentially activated during β-cell development. Two transcription factors, Pax 4 (paired box gene 4) and Arx (arista-less-related homeobox protein) are antagonistic in their actions, similarly to two light switches in different areas of a room that, when flicked, can turn each other on or off. Pax and Arx can be modulated by histone modification in order to influence the β-cell (Collombat et al. 2007). One of the most important genes in the β-cell is the insulin gene, and the insulin gene promoter has sites for hyperacetylation and other sites for hypermethylation in order to regulate the β-cell insulin gene. Under high-glucose conditions, such as in diabetes, changes in histone acetylation have been shown to regulate β-cell survival and function (see Johnson and Evans-Molina 2015 for a more thorough discussion of these changes).

Finally, epigenetic changes in response to the environment have been documented in utero. Intrauterine growth restriction (IUGR) results from poor maternal nutrition. IUGR offspring are likely to develop obesity and type 2 diabetes, with epigenetics playing a role in this phenomenon (Barker et al. 1993; Simmons et al. 2001). Even though this work was done in rats, it is believed that this may also occur in other organisms, including humans. This is why prenatal care is so important for mothers and their children. It is not only the mother that is responsible for epigenetic changes, but a high-fat diet in fathers has been shown to lead to β-cell dysfunction and altered expression of many genes in the pancreas regulating metabolism in their children (Ng et al. 2010).

GENOMICS, EPIGENETICS, AND ENVIRONMENT IN MENTAL ILLNESSES

Twin studies have revealed profound facts about the relationships between genomics, epigenetics, and environmental influences in the diagnosis of mental illness. According to the World Health Organization (WHO), 40% of the medical disabilities of U.S. and Canadian people aged 15–44 consist of mental illnesses. Twin studies have demonstrated the high level of heritability of diseases such as autism, bipolar disorder, and schizophrenia (Insel and Wang 2010). Candidate genes and alleles identified from GWAS have only been able to explain a small fraction of the heritability of these mental diseases. So what is the reason for this heritability? One of the possibilities comes from the discovery of large structural changes in the genes, specifically different numbers of copies such as deletions and duplications in the genes, called copy number variants (Figure 3.3), which are more than ten-fold more common in individuals with autism or schizophrenia (Sebat et al. 2007; Walsh et al. 2008). Many of these affected genes appear to be involved in brain development. Within families, schizophrenia with a particular copy variant may be found in one person, while the same difference leads to bipolar disorder in another family member and attention deficit/hyperactivity disorder in yet another (Sebat et al. 2007; Walsh et al. 2008).

The genetics of mental illness may really be the genetics of brain development, with different outcomes being possible depending on biological and environmental influences and epigenetics (Sebat et al. 2007; Walsh et al. 2008). For instance, a rare copy number variant detected in autism deletes the oxytocin receptor gene. In other individuals with autism, epigenetic changes, in particular DNA methylation of the CpG islands known to regulate gene expression, appear to silence the oxytocin receptor gene (Gregory et al. 2009). Oxytocin is a very

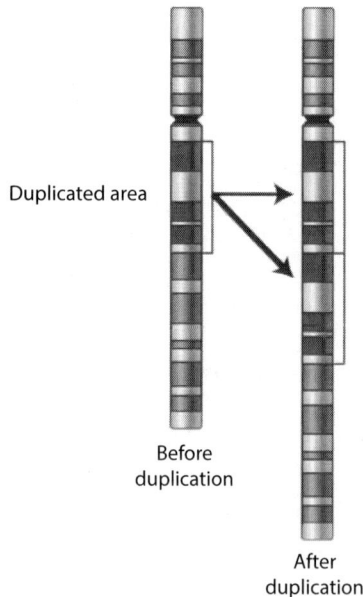

Duplicated area

Before duplication

After duplication

Figure 3.3 Gene duplication and copy number variants. In the diagram, only one section of the DNA is copied in order to create a structural variation in the DNA. However, genomes in some individuals can have many different numbers of copies, such as duplications or even deletions of sections of the DNA on a chromosome, and these are called copy number variants. (Courtesy of the National Human Genome Research Institute.)

interesting hormone that is produced by the hypothalamus and is considered to be a neuromodulator in sexual reproduction, childbirth, and social recognition and bonding. In fact, it is called the "bonding hormone" in human interactions. Thus, genomics, epigenetics, and the environment appear to interact in order to promote the risk for particular mental illnesses, and even affect social interactions.

In grade school, I have a vivid memory of studying the raging scientific controversy of Lamarck versus Darwin, and who was correct in his view of inheritance. Jean-Baptist Lamarck (1744–1829) was a French biologist who put forth the evolutionary theory that the main mechanism for diversity in animal and plant life was due to adaptation during the lifetime of the organism in response to environmental influences, which could be inherited and influence the offspring of the next generation.

What shocked me as a child was the life story of Paul Kammerer (1880–1926), an Austrian biologist and follower of Lamarck. Kammerer performed an experiment with midwife toads that normally lived on land but were forced in the laboratory to live in water over a span of several generations. (He also performed similar types of experiments with salamanders and other reptiles with the same findings.) With time, these midwife toads developed black nuptial pads on their feet so that they had more traction during mating in the water. The prehistoric ancestors of these toads had these pads, and Kammerer had shown that these toads could reacquire these characteristics due to adaptation to the environment (Schmuck 2000). On tour with these new findings, somehow someone exchanged the toads and placed black ink pads on the toad's feet, which lead to Kammerer being disgraced. Even though other scientists had previously verified his finding by close examination of these toads and via photographs, Dr. G.K. Noble, Curator of Reptiles at the American Museum of American History, published in the scientific journal *Nature* that Dr. Kammerer had falsified his results (Noble 1926). Six weeks after the *Nature* publication, Dr. Kammerer committed suicide.

The true story of Kammerer made a tremendous impression on me, perhaps due to the fact that this was my first exposure to suicide. I never could wholeheartedly believe that "the survival of the fittest" was the sole driving force of genetic changes as Charles Darwin had so eloquently written in his great treatise, *The Origin of Species*, published in 1859. In 2009, the developmental biologist Alexander Vargas suggested that the inheritance of acquired traits that Kammerer had found with the midwife toads could be explained by epigenetics and DNA methylation (Pennisi 2009; Vargas 2009). I believe that Lamarck, Kammerer, and Darwin were all partly correct about inheritance, and it is terribly unfortunate that politics, jealousy, and bias can obscure scientific discoveries, cause someone's death, and cover up scientific findings and the truth.

miRNAs, siRNAs, AND piRNAs

In the plant and animal kingdoms, siRNAs and miRNAs are broadly distributed and affect the expression of many genes, mostly by silencing them (Cathew and Sontheimer 2009). miRNAs are regulators of endogenous genes, while siRNAs respond to foreign nucleic acids such as viruses. The foreign nucleic acid can also be a transposon, a gene that is able to jump to different regions of the genome and is thought to be a remnant of a viral or parasitic infection that occurred to our ancestors. Alternatively, the foreign DNA can be a transgene, a gene that is inserted into the genome. Both miRNAs and siRNAs have precursors that are double stranded and bind to Argonaute proteins in order to exert their effects. These double-stranded precursor RNAs have long sequences and need to be cleaved by specific enzymes: first by Drosha with the help of DGCR8, and then they are further cleaved by Dicer to form the mature miRNA or siRNA. Then, both RNAs activate the RNA-induced silencing complex (RISC), which finds the complementary target mRNA sequence to be cleaved and inactivated (Figure 3.4). This biological process, in which RNA molecules inhibit gene expression by causing the destruction of specific mRNAs, is collectively called RNAi.

miRNAs are small RNAs, being about 20–24 nucleotides long, which bind to the end (3′ untranslated region [UTR]) of mRNA. mRNAs are responsible for specifying the amino acid sequence of a protein, a product of gene expression of the DNA. miRNAs are promiscuous, meaning that one specific miRNA can bind to many mRNAs and affect many proteins. Usually, they repress gene expression by degrading the specific mRNA or inhibiting its translation into a protein. More than 2555 miRNA sequences have been found in humans, and they affect 60% of protein-coding genes (Ebert and Sharp 2012; Sethi et al. 2014). In other words, miRNAs play a role in virtually every cellular process in our body, including cell proliferation, differentiation, and apoptosis (cell death). A typical miRNA will only cause a small reduction in a protein's level and many miRNAs can be deleted without causing a change in characteristics/phenotype. So why are they needed in us or other organisms such as plants, invertebrates, and other vertebrates?

A theory regarding the need for many miRNAs comes from the concept that miRNAs can cause "robustness" in biological processes (Ebert and Sharp 2012). By having different expression profiles in different tissues, even if these tissues originate from the same cell progenitor, miRNAs are able to modulate development by repressing transcripts from a previous stage in development, and so contribute to the appropriate development of cells and tissues. miRNAs have also been suggested to act as "buffers" against variation in gene expression, since they can modulate the results of gene expression (i.e., protein levels) without transcription being up- or down-regulated, and so affect different cell activities. Therefore, some miRNA roles can be likened to dimmers on your light switch that allow you to change the lighting without interrupting the flow of electricity running through the wires in your home.

Other miRNAs do not appear to change the phenotype of a cell, tissue, or animal if they are deleted, but if that cell, tissue, or animal is challenged by an event either externally or internally, then their role becomes clear in allowing

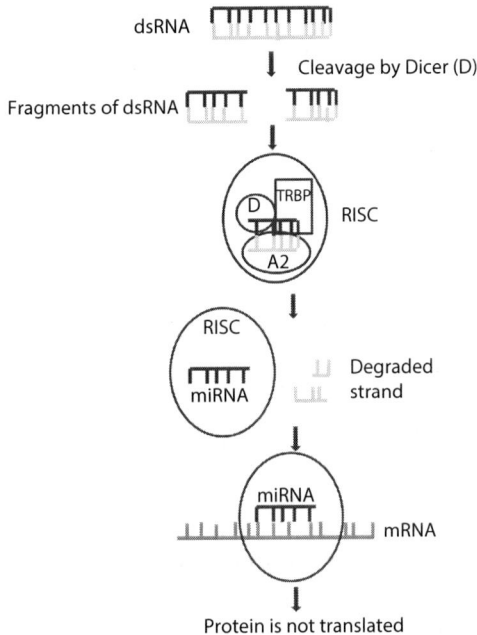

Figure 3.4 RNA interference. Both miRNAs and siRNAs have precursors that are double-stranded RNAs (dsRNAs) and are cleaved by Dicer (D) to form the mature miRNA or siRNA. Then, either miRNAs or siRNAs can activate the RNA-induced silencing complex (RISC). RISC allows the loading of dsRNA fragments generated by the endonuclease D onto Argonaute 2 (A2) with the help of the trans-activation response RNA-binding protein (TRBP). This complex finds the complementary target mRNA sequence to be cleaved and inactivated. miRNAs silence the translation of proteins by mRNA through base pairing with the mRNA. The nucleotide sequence of the miRNA does not need to pair exactly with the nucleotide sequence of the mRNA in order to block translation. The mRNA molecule is silenced by one or more of the following processes: cleavage of the mRNA; destabilizing the mRNA; and less efficient translation of the mRNA into proteins.

adaptation or maladaptation to a new situation for survival. In a myriad of diverse responses to the environment, miRNAs allow a cell, tissue, or animal to survive a change in environment while other cells, tissues, or animals are unable to do so. This change results in the survival or adaptation of only a few organisms, creating diversity. Robustness in a group of people or animals can allow them to be strong and adaptive (i.e., "robust") in response to changes in their environment. However, the presence of miRNA, affecting all of our cells' activities, makes it difficult to know what will be the expression of a gene in a lifetime, once that gene or mutation is identified from genomic screening (i.e., knowledge of which genes and mutations you have does not tell you which diseases you may or may not develop).

piRNAs are primarily found in animals and are most important in the germline, where they repress gene expression. Little is known about these RNAs, but it appears that they are single stranded and also bind to members of specific Piwi-associated proteins, thus differing from miRNAs and siRNAs. The wide variation in piRNA sequences and functions across many different species makes it difficult to determine their exact function. However, piRNAs do act in both epigenetic and post-transcriptional gene silencing, particularly in germline cells, such as in spermatogenesis, and they are critical to the development of the human embryo.

miRNAs AND CANCER

A pitfall in using genomics as a basis for disease diagnosis is that miRNAs can alter disease expression such that you will not know if you will ever manifest the disease in your lifetime. In addition, miRNAs can have an adverse effect when co-opted in cancer. On the other hand, miRNAs may be promising as therapeutic tools for determining the stage and prognosis for cancer patients. Can miRNAs be used to personalize medical treatment? Relatively recently (i.e., in 2002), the first report of miRNAs in cancer was published, with miR-15 and miR-16 being shown to be deleted in most people with chronic lymphocytic leukemia (CLL) (Calin et al. 2002). A study of 328 human miRNAs in patients with breast cancer has identified miR-210 as having such high prognostic value that finding overexpression of miR-210 alone had the same prognostic value as a 76-gene mRNA signature test. Its overexpression was associated with increased risk of breast cancer recurrence (Rothé et al. 2011). Subsequently it was found that these miRNAs are tumor suppressors since they affect BCL2, an oncogene that encodes a protein that is important in cell survival (Cimmino et al. 2005). The same group of investigators as those who discovered the first miRNAs in CLL has gone on to identify groups of miRNAs in patients with CLL that can predict disease severity and progression (Calin et al. 2002). Thus, miRNAs are being studied for their prognostic value in specific cancers with the hope that these patients can then be targeted for different treatments (Kong et al. 2012).

In contrast, miR-21 is overexpressed in most cancers (e.g., breast cancer, lung cancer, colorectal cancer, glioblastoma, leukemia, and lymphoma) (Kong et al. 2012). Many of these cancers are dependent on the expression of miR-21, which has become a target for cancer research. However, miRNAs are promiscuous, as was said previously, and they affect many cell processes, especially normal processes, so it becomes a challenge to target only the bad miR-21.

Another advantage of miRNAs is that some of them are also found in body fluids, which would allow scientists to easily test these fluids for early signs or biomarkers of various diseases (Brase et al. 2010). Human plasma contains about 350 different miRNAs and it would be helpful to use these miRNAs as markers for diseases, especially cancer, but there has been little consensus between studies regarding which miRNAs are the best markers for a particular cancer (Witwer 2015). In one study, miR-195 and lethal-7a (let-7a) miRNA were higher in breast cancer patients, and these miRNAs decreased after surgery (Heneghan et al. 2010). It is hoped that miRNAs will have therapeutic potential for many diseases, including breast cancer, so that a more personalized approach to disease staging can be developed in order to determine the best treatment.

miRNAs AND HEPATITIS C

In addition to their diagnostic potential, the delivery of miRNAs may be used to treat other diseases, including hepatitis C. A therapy for hepatitis C that is being developed contains miR-122. One problem with miRNAs is that they have low stability in vivo, so they are cleared from the circulation very rapidly. Scientists are trying to develop nanoparticles with attached miRNAs that would allow the miRNAs to remain in the circulation for longer and enter only into tumors, since tumor blood vessels are known to have larger pores than normal vessels (Heneghan et al. 2010). This approach requires biomaterial scientists to use their knowledge of materials and then, with the knowledge from medicine, biology, chemistry, tissue engineering, and other scientists, devise novel therapeutics. Biomaterial scientists have devised methods such as the use of locked nucleic acid (LNA) to increase the stability of LNA–RNA duplexes to deliver miRNA. This technology was used to target miR-122 for the treatment of people with hepatitis C. miR-122 is found predominantly in the liver and is an essential miRNA for hepatitis C virus replication. A miRNA-based drug trial in chimpanzees used LNA to remove miR-122 and stop infections. Once-a-week treatments for 12 weeks in chronically infected chimpanzees led to a reduction in viral load in the liver and serum. After treatments were stopped, these declines were maintained for 13 weeks and liver appearance in histological sections improved (Lanford et al. 2010). This study led to the first preliminary clinical trials of miRNAs in people (Janssen et al. 2013), and this approach appears to be promising as a new therapy for hepatitis C infections.

A close friend of mine was diagnosed with hepatitis C more than 20 years ago. His disease is not active—at least that is what he believes—and he has hesitated to go for therapy because the present therapy of hepatitis C, alpha interferon, can have many side effects. Alpha interferons have been used since the late 1980s in the treatment of chronic hepatitis C. In fact, we recently visited someone who went through this therapy twice (as it did not work the first time). He was cured, but he experienced severe neurological damage to his legs and has cognition deficits. He had to leave his job and stay at home, where he goes a bit stir crazy, and as he cannot drive well, it is hard for him to find another job. My close friend is now considering the new drug Sovaldi (sofosbuvir in combination with ribavirin) for his hepatitis C, because it seems to have fewer side effects and a better cure rate. However, it costs $1,000 per pill each day or $84,000 for a typical course of treatment. The drug inhibits the RNA polymerase that the hepatitis C virus uses to replicate its RNA. Thus, present therapies have their issues, and it is hoped that miRNA therapies may be a better solution.

The study of miRNAs and their impacts on gene expression is a young field of science, similarly to other areas of epigenetics. Epigenetics complicates the analysis of risk factors and outcomes of any personal genomic data and complicates the goals of personalized medicine. However, as a field of science, it is very exciting and should provide novel approaches for understanding disease progression and perhaps targeting the cells involved in disease processes.

REFERENCES

Barker, DJ, CN Hales, CH Fall, C Osmond, K Phipps, and PM Clark. 1993. Type 2 (non-insulin-dependent) diabetes mellitus, hypertension and hyperlipidaemia (syndrome X): Relation to reduced fetal growth. *Diabetologia* 36(1):62–7.

Brase, JC, D Wuttig, R Kuner, and H Sültmann. 2010. Serum microRNAs as non-invasive biomarkers for cancer. *Mol Cancer* 9:306.

Calin, GA, CD Dumitru, M Shimizu et al. 2002. Frequent deletions and down-regulation of micro-RNA genes miR15 and miR16 at 13q14 in chronic lymphocytic leukemia. *Proc Natl Acad Sci USA* 99(24):15524–9.

Cathew, RW and EJ Sontheimer. 2009. Origins and mechanism of miRNA and siRNAs. *Cell* 136:642–55.

Cimmino, A, GA Calin, M Fabbri et al. 2005. miR-15 and miR-16 induce apoptosis by targeting BCL2. *Proc Natl Acad Sci USA* 102(39):13944–9.

Collombat, P, J Hecksher-Sørensen, J Krull, J Berger, D Riedel, PL Herrera, P Serup, and A Mansouri. 2007. Embryonic endocrine pancreas and mature beta cells acquire alpha and PP cell phenotypes upon Arx misexpression. *J Clin Invest* 117(4):961–70.

Ebert, MS and PA Sharp. 2012. Roles for microRNAs in conferring robustness to biological processes. *Cell* 149(3):515–24.

Fraga, MF, E Ballestar, MF Paz et al. 2005. Epigenetic differences arise during the lifetime of monozygotic twins. *Proc Natl Acad Sci USA* 102:10604–9.

Gregory, SG, JJ Connelly, AJ Towers et al. 2009. Genomic and epigenetic evidence for oxytocin receptor deficiency in autism. *BMC Med* 7:62.

Guariguata, L, DR Whiting, I Hambleton, J Beagley, U Linnenkamp, and JE Shaw. 2014. Global estimates of diabetes prevalence for 2013 and projections for 2035. *Diabetes Res Clin Pract* 103(2):137–49.

Guénard, F, Y Deshaies, K Cianflone, JG Kral, P Marceau, and MC Vohl. 2013. Differential methylation in glucoregulatory genes of offspring born before vs. after maternal gastrointestinal bypass surgery. *Proc Natl Acad Sci USA* 110(28):11439–44.

Heneghan, HM, N Miller, and MJ Kerin. 2010. Circulating miRNA signatures: Promising prognostic tools for cancer. *J Clin Oncol* 28:e573–4.

Insel, TR and PS Wang. 2010. Rethinking mental illness. *JAMA* 303(19):1970–1.

Janssen, HL, S Kauppinen, and MR Hodges. 2013. HCV infection and miravirsen. *N Engl J Med* 369(9):878.

Johnson, JS and C Evans-Molina. 2015. Translational implications of the β-cell epigenome in diabetes mellitus. *Transl Res* 165(1):91–101.

Kong, YW, D Ferland-McCollough, TJ Jackson, and M Bushell. 2012. MicroRNAs in cancer management. *Lancet Oncol* 13(6):e249–58.

Lanford, RE, ES Hildebrandt-Eriksen, A Petri, R Persson, M Lindow, ME Munk, S Kauppinen, and H Ørum. 2010. Therapeutic silencing of microRNA-122 in primates with chronic hepatitis C virus infection. *Science* 327(5962):198–201.

Ng, SF, RC Lin, DR Laybutt, R Barres, JA Owens, and MJ Morris. 2010. Chronic high-fat diet in fathers programs β-cell dysfunction in female rat offspring. *Nature* 467(7318):963–6.

Noble, GK 1926. Kammerer's alytes. *Nature* 118(2962):209–11.

Patti, ME. 2013. Reducing maternal weight improves offspring metabolism and alters (or modulates) methylation. *Proc Natl Acad Sci USA* 110(32):12859–60.

Pennisi, E. 2009. The case of the midwife toad: Fraud or epigenetics? *Science* 325(5945):1194–5.

Rothé, F, M Ignatiadis, C Chaboteaux et al. 2011. Global microRNA expression profiling identifies miR-210 associated with tumor proliferation, invasion and poor clinical outcome in breast cancer. *PLoS One* 6(6):e20980.

Schmuck, T. 2000. The midwife toad and human progress. Hofrichter, R. (ed.). *Amphibians: The World of Frogs, Toads, Salamanders and Newts*. New York: Firefly. pp. 212–3.

Sebat, J, B Lakshmi, D Malhotra et al. 2007. Strong association of *de novo* copy number mutations with autism. *Science* 316(5823):445–9.

Sethi, S, S Ali, S Sethi, and FH Sarkar. 2014. MicroRNAs in personalized cancer therapy. *Clin Genet* 86(1):68–73.

Simmons, RA, LJ Templeton, and SJ Gertz. 2001. Intrauterine growth retardation leads to the development of type 2 diabetes. *Diabetes* 50:2279–86.

Temple, IK and JP Shield. 2010. 6q24 transient neonatal diabetes. *Rev Endocr Metab Disord* 11(3):199–204.

Vargas, AO. 2009. Did Paul Kammerer discover epigenetic inheritance? A modern look at the controversial midwife toad experiments. *J Exp Zool B Mol Dev Evol* 312(7):667–78.

Volkmar, M, S Dedeurwaerder, DA Cunha et al. 2012. DNA methylation profiling identifies epigenetic dysregulation in pancreatic islets from type 2 diabetic patients. *EMBO J* 31(6):1405–26.

Walsh, T, JM McClellan, SE McCarthy et al. 2008. Rare structural variants disrupt multiple genes in neurodevelopmental pathways in schizophrenia. *Science* 320(5875):539–43.

Wei, FY, K Nagashima, T Ohshima et al. 2005. Cdk5-dependent regulation of glucose-stimulated insulin secretion. *Nat Med* 11(10):1104–8.

Weksberg, R, C Shuman, O Caluseriu, et al. 2002. Discordant KCNQ1OT1 imprinting in sets of monozygotic twins discordant for Beckwith–Wiedemann syndrome. *Hum Mol Genet* 11(11):1317–25.

Witwer, KW. 2015. Circulating microRNA biomarker studies: Pitfalls and potential solutions. *Clin Chem* 61(1):56–63.

4

Integrative medicine: Nutrition and exercise

How important is your own nutrition to you? What roles do nutrition and exercising play in preventing disease?

Nutrition is a part of integrative medicine, and its importance needs to be highlighted and supported. The Consortium of Academic Health Centers for Integrative Medicine defines integrative medicine as "the practice of medicine that reaffirms the importance of the relationship between practitioner and patient, focuses on the whole person, is informed by evidence, and makes use of all appropriate therapeutic approaches, healthcare professionals and disciplines to achieve optimal health and healing." Many of the topics in integrative medicine are part of the domain of complementary and alternative medicine (CAM), but the CAM term is not used as often. Instead, integrative medicine encompasses only those therapies of CAM that are based on evidence from strong scientific studies to support their use as therapeutic tools.

Even though nutrition is basic to human existence, it has not been incorporated readily into the armamentarium of physicians dealing with patients' health issues, and thus it can be considered part of integrative medicine. Often, we do not get advice or are asked about our diet until we have a medical problem. Why is diet ignored, even when there is a medical issue? Why is what you eat not discussed when you are young/healthy? Early changes in diet can prevent the development of diseases such as atherosclerosis, diabetes, or other diseases that are influenced by diet.

We have touched briefly in previous chapters on some nutritional effects on disease outcomes. In the proteomics chapter, obesity and losing weight can have a positive impact on cancer progression and outcomes. In the same chapter, cholesterol levels were shown to play a role in cardiovascular disease, and we know that intake of high levels of fat and carbohydrates in processed foods increases our risk for heart disease and diabetes. Nutrition and exercise levels during childhood can impact bone mass and the chance of developing osteoporosis later in life, as was shown in the genomics chapter. Nutrition affects every aspect of our lives and can influence the development and outcomes of disease. However, many nutritional effects take time to accrue, and in general require long-term changes in lifestyle. A more comprehensive analysis of nutrition with health and disease outcomes requires a book to cover all of its aspects, and in this chapter we will only cover a few topics in order to illustrate nutrition's profound effects on our health.

HEALTHY DIET

The Nutrition Committee of the American Heart Association has suggestions for a healthy cardiovascular system. These guidelines should be followed by the majority of normal people (Krauss et al. 2001).

A diet that contains a variety of foods from all food categories is best, with an emphasis on fruits and vegetables (especially dark green, deep orange, or yellow vegetables), legumes (the most common being different types of beans) and nuts, fish, poultry, and lean meats (Figure 4.1). At least six or more servings of grain products, especially whole grains, are recommended each day. Foods that are high in starches are better for you than foods with lots of sugar. Due to the cardiovascular benefits of eating fish, the consumption of at least two fish servings per week is recommended. Blood pressure can be reduced by consuming vegetables, fruits, and low-fat dairy products, as well as limiting salt intake (<6 g/day) and limiting alcohol to no more than 2 drinks per day for men and 1 drink per day for women. Drinking plenty of water is healthy, while sodas are unhealthy. Butter and oils such as olive and canola oils are recommended, while we should avoid trans fats in processed foods. Finally, a healthy body weight is beneficial for maintaining normal blood pressure and for improving your cardiovascular risk. Knowing your height and weight can give you your body mass index (BMI), as there are many calculators online that can tell you your BMI by just providing your weight and height.

BMI

BMI is an old concept that was developed by Adolphe Quetelet in the first half of the nineteenth century. BMI is defined as an individual's body mass divided by the square of their height—with the value being given in units of kg/m^2.

$$BMI = \frac{Mass\ (kg)}{(Height\ (m))^2}$$

$$BMI = \frac{Mass\ (pounds)}{(Height\ (inches))^2} \times 703$$

With this calculator, these are the guidelines for BMI:
Underweight = <18.5
Normal weight = 18.5–24.9
Overweight = 25–29.9
Obesity = BMI of 30 or greater

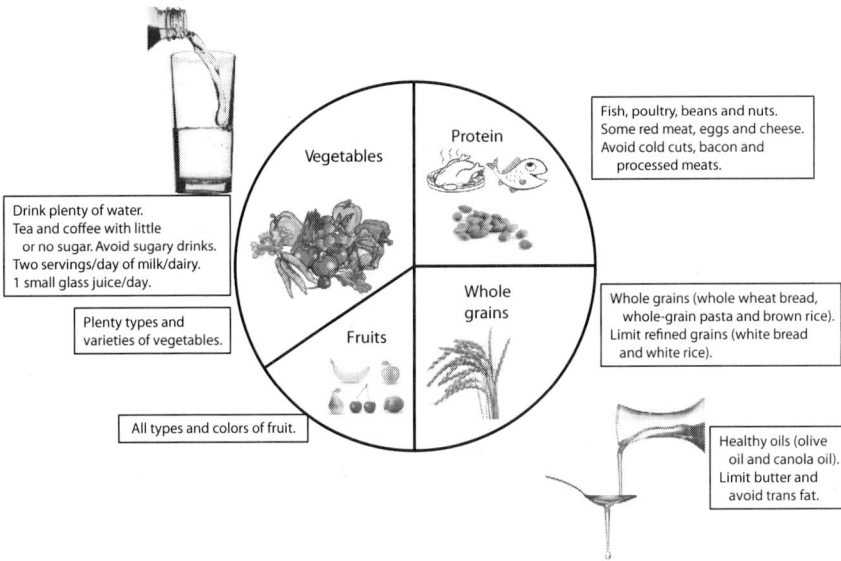

Figure 4.1 Schematic of what foods and drinks should comprise healthy eating for adults. It is highly recommended that vegetables and fruits of multiple colors and varieties make up half of the foods that are ingested. Potatoes do not count, since they have a negative impact on blood sugar. Fish, chicken, beans, and nuts are all healthy protein sources. Red meat should be limited, and processed meats such as bacon should be avoided. Whole and intact grains (whole wheat, barley, quinoa, oats, and brown rice) and foods made with them, such as whole wheat pasta, are healthy. White bread, white rice, and other refined grains have a more negative effect on blood sugar. Sugary drinks are also unhealthy, and drinking several glasses of water per day is recommended. Milk/dairy products and juices should also be limited. Healthy plant oils such as olive, canola, soy, sunflower, peanut, and corn oils are recommended, while partially hydrogenated oils should be avoided, since they contain unhealthy trans fats. The relative sizes of the pie shapes in the diagram reflect the approximate proportions of each food group, but do not reflect calorie intake or number of servings each day. Individuals' calorie and nutrient needs vary based on age, gender, body size, and level of activity.

VITAMINS

One area of nutrition is vitamins: vitamin A, C, E, K, and different B vitamins (Table 4.1). Vitamins are essential for normal growth and development, and once a child reaches adulthood, vitamins help to maintain cells, tissues, and organs. If there is serious deficiency in one or more vitamins during child development, then permanent damage can occur. Vitamins enable us to produce the chemical energy we need from the food we eat. These nutrients contribute to the healthy development and maintenance of skin, bone, and muscle. Most of our vitamins are obtained from the food we eat, but a few, like vitamin K, are produced by microorganisms in our intestine.

Table 4.1 Vitamins and their sources in food

Vitamin	Chemical name	Food source
A	Retinol, retinal, four carotenoids, including β-carotene	Liver, yellow and orange fruits, leafy vegetables, carrots, squash, pumpkin, fish, milk, soy milk
B1	Thiamine	Oatmeal, brown rice, vegetables, liver, pork, eggs
B2	Riboflavin	Dairy products, bananas, green beans, asparagus
B3	Niacin, niacinamide	Meat, fish, eggs, many vegetables, mushrooms, tree nuts
B5	Pantothenic acid	Meat, broccoli, avocado
B6	Pyridoxine, pyridoxamine, pyridoxal	Meat, vegetables, bananas, tree nuts
B7	Biotin	Raw egg yolk, liver, leafy green vegetables, peanuts
B9	Folic acid, foline acid	Leafy vegetables, pasta, bread, cereal, liver
B12	Cyanocobalamin, hydroxycobalamin, methylcobalamin	Meat
C	Ascorbic acid	Many fruits and vegetables, liver
D	Cholecalciferol (D3), ergocalciferol (D2)	Fish, eggs, liver, mushrooms
E	Tocopherols, tocotrienols	Many fruits and vegetables, nuts and seeds
K	Phylloquinone, menaquinone	Leafy green vegetables, egg yolks, liver

There has been conflicting evidence on the benefits of vitamin supplementation and the ability of vitamins to reduce risk of disease. Of course, vitamins are necessary for many biological processes in our bodies, and most vitamins are ingested through a normal diet. The clearest example of the benefit from vitamins comes from the scientific literature on vitamin D, which helps the body use calcium and phosphorus for strong bones and teeth. Most of the vitamin D for our bodies is obtained by exposure of the skin to sunlight, but it can also be acquired from food and dietary supplements. Our skin synthesizes cholecalciferol from cholesterol in the skin, and then further modifications in the liver and kidney produce vitamin D. Vitamin D is often called the "sunshine vitamin." Some studies have suggested that higher intake of vitamin D can reduce the risk of colorectal cancer (Woolcott et al. 2010; Ma et al. 2011), but not other cancers (Gandini et al. 2011). It is unclear whether vitamin D reduces the risk of other cancers, including breast and prostate cancers. Scientific evidence with cancer cells and tumors in mice has shown that vitamin D slows or prevents the development of cancer by decreasing cancer cell growth and increasing cancer cell death (apoptosis), reducing tumor blood vessel formation (angiogenesis), and promoting cell differentiation (Holt et al. 2002; Moreno et al. 2005; Deeb et al. 2007; Thorne and Campbell 2008).

The Institute of Medicine (IOM) of the National Academies has developed the following recommendations on the daily intake of vitamin D, assuming minimal sun exposure (Ross et al. 2011):

- For those between 1 and 70 years of age, including women who are pregnant or lactating, the recommended dietary allowance (RDA) is 15 µg per day or 600 international units (IU) (1 µg = 40 IU).
- For those 71 years or older, the RDA is 20 µg per day (800 IU per day).
- For infants, the IOM could not determine a recommended dose due to a lack of data. However, the IOM set an adequate intake level of 10 µg per day (400 IU per day).

More than 80% of Americans have adequate vitamin D levels in their blood, according to the National Health and Nutrition Examination Survey. However, improving calcium and vitamin D nutritional status substantially reduced all-cancer risk in postmenopausal women (Lappe et al. 2007).

It is also important to realize that excessive intake of any vitamin can cause toxic effects. Too much vitamin D can cause increased levels of calcium that can lead to calcinosis—the depositing of calcium salt in soft tissues such as the lungs or kidneys—or hypercalcemia—high blood levels of calcium. Another approach to reducing the risk of cancer is to eat more vegetables and fruits, which have been found to reduce bladder cancer in women and also to reduce the risk of other cancers (Park et al. 2013).

> My cousin's husband had occlusion of his arteries with plaques and had to have a stent placed in some of his blood vessels. Stents are small, expandable tubes that are used to treat narrowed or weakened arteries in the body so that the vessels remain opened for blood flow. His doctor has cautioned him against taking too many vitamin D pills, since this approach might increase calcification and the problems with his arteries. Again, personalized care for my cousin's husband showed that he should watch his vitamin D levels due to his cardiovascular disease. The upper limit for vitamin D intake is 100 µg per day (4000 IU).

MINERALS IN OUR DIET

Minerals and other nutrients also have an impact on health and are important to consider in a healthy diet. Table 4.2 lists the following minerals found in food and their importance for bodily function: Sodium, chloride, potassium, calcium,

Table 4.2 Major minerals found in our food that are essential for health

Mineral	Function	Sources
Sodium	Proper body fluid balance, nerve transmission, and muscle contraction	Table salt, soy sauce, large amounts in processed foods, small amounts in milk, breads, vegetables, and unprocessed meats
Chloride	Proper body fluid balance and stomach acid	Table salt, soy sauce, large amounts in processed foods, small amounts in milk, meats, breads, and vegetables
Potassium	Proper body fluid balance, nerve transmission, and muscle contraction	Meats, milk, fresh fruits and vegetables, whole grains, and legumes
Calcium	Bone and dental health, helps relax and contract muscles, nerve functioning, blood clotting, blood pressure regulation, and the immune system	Milk and milk products, canned fish with bones (salmon and sardines), fortified tofu and fortified soy milk, greens (broccoli and mustard greens), and legumes
Phosphorus	Bone and dental health, cell function, and maintains acid–base balance	Meat, fish, poultry, eggs, milk, and processed foods (including soda)
Magnesium	Bones, muscle contraction, nerve transmission, the immune system, and is needed for making protein	Nuts and seeds, legumes, leafy green vegetables, seafood, chocolate, artichokes, and "hard" drinking water
Sulfur	Protein molecules	In foods as part of protein, meats, poultry, fish, eggs, milk, legumes, and nuts

Source: Modified from http://www.emedicinehealth.com/minerals_their_functions_and_sources-health/article_em.htm

phosphorus, magnesium, and sulfur. Trace metals are shown in Table 4.3 and they too have essential functions. Other trace minerals that are important in tiny amounts are nickel, sodium, vanadium, and cobalt.

Elemental iron has important functions for all cells and facilitates cell growth and metabolism. Iron can participate in enzymatic reactions due to its ability to gain and lose electrons. One of these classes of reactions in the cell is the ability for iron to participate in free-radical generation. Among these reactions is one that can produce hydroxyl radicals that can damage lipids,

Table 4.3 Trace minerals (microminerals) that are important for health

Mineral	Function	Sources
Iron	In hemoglobin of red blood cells that carries oxygen in the body; energy metabolism; although iron is considered a trace metal, somewhat more is needed than for other trace minerals	Red meats, fish, poultry, shellfish (especially clams), egg yolks, legumes, dried fruits, dark, leafy greens, iron-enriched breads and cereals, and fortified cereals
Zinc	In enzymes; needed for making proteins and genetic material; taste perception; wound healing; normal fetal development; production of sperm; normal growth and sexual maturation; immune system health	Meats, fish, poultry, leavened whole grains, and vegetables
Iodine	In thyroid hormone, which helps regulate growth, development, and metabolism	Seafood, foods grown in iodine-rich soil, iodized salt, bread, and dairy products
Selenium	Antioxidant	Meats, seafood, and grains
Copper	In enzymes; needed for iron metabolism	Legumes, nuts and seeds, whole grains, meats, and drinking water
Manganese	In enzymes	Widespread in foods, especially plants
Fluoride	Formation of bones and teeth; helps prevent tooth decay	Drinking water (either fluoridated or naturally containing fluoride), fish, and most teas
Chromium	Works with insulin to regulate blood sugar (glucose) levels	Unrefined foods, liver, brewer's yeast, whole grains, nuts, and cheeses
Molybdenum	In some enzymes	Legumes, breads and grains, leafy green vegetables, milk, and liver

Source: Modified from http://www.emedicinehealth.com/minerals_their_functions_and_sources-health/article_em.htm

proteins, and even DNA. Thus, it is surmised that iron may also be able to modify DNA, cause mutations, and contribute to cancer. However, normal iron levels are crucial for our bodies and cells to function. A comprehensive review article has been published on this topic by scientists at my institution (Torti and Torti 2013).

> The article on iron led me to think about why I developed breast cancer. No one in my family had ever had breast cancer, to my knowledge. Due to my hemangiomas and the ensuing internal bleeding problem I have had since I was 12 years old, I have had to take large doses of iron simply to maintain my hematocrit. Hematocrit is measured by a blood test and is the volume percentage of red blood cells in the blood. It is normally about 45% for men and 40% for women. Iron is essential for making red blood cells and for their function. I have often been anemic, falling below the normal 40%, so my doctors prescribed a large dose of iron. All my life, I was monitored with blood tests to make sure that my ferritin levels did not go too high and that my hematocrit was in the normal range. Ferritin is an intracellular protein that stores iron so that it can be used later by the body. Testing for ferritin in the blood was a way to measure the amount of iron in the blood. I do not think a test ever came back too high. I was always on the low side. I wonder if taking iron every day for most of my life contributed to my breast cancer.

METABOLIC SYNDROME, CHOLESTEROL, LOW-DENSITY LIPOPROTEINS, HIGH-DENSITY LIPOPROTEINS, AND BLOOD PRESSURE

One of the biggest problems in the United States is obesity and the development of metabolic syndrome. Nutrition plays a critical role in this disease. Metabolic syndrome is a disorder of energy storage and utilization, and is diagnosed based on someone having at least three of the following five criteria: increased abdominal fat (i.e., increased central body girth); elevated blood pressure; increased fasting glucose levels in blood; high serum triglycerides (a blood lipid); and low high-density cholesterol (HDL) levels (Table 4.4).

Reducing "bad" low-density lipoprotein (LDL) cholesterol and increasing "good" HDL cholesterol may lower the risk of heart disease depending on the present levels in your blood, which can only be determined by a doctor from a blood test (Figure 4.2). Cholesterol is a wax-like substance that is found in cells, especially cell membranes, but it is also found in the bloodstream attached to these lipoproteins. LDL carries cholesterol throughout the body, and delivers it to different organs and tissues. However, if LDL is in excess, then LDL circulates repeatedly in the bloodstream, and will start to build up in blood vessels by forming plaques that narrow the vessels, causing atherosclerosis. These plaques are composed of white blood cells due to inflammation, cholesterol, and

Table 4.4 Metabolic syndrome as defined by the American Heart Association and the National Heart, Lung, and Blood Institute

Large waist size	For men: 40 inches or larger
	For women: 35 inches or larger
Cholesterol: high triglycerides	150 mg/dL or higher or using a cholesterol medicine
Cholesterol: low good cholesterol (high-density lipoprotein)	For men: less than 40 mg/dL
	For women: less than 50 mg/dL or using a cholesterol medicine for both sexes
High blood pressure	Having a blood pressure of >135/85 mm Hg or using a high-blood pressure medicine
Blood sugar: high fasting glucose level	100 mg/dL or higher

Note: Having at least three of the five risk factors listed above leads to a diagnosis of metabolic syndrome.

triglycerides, along with calcium and other crystallized minerals. Eventually, plaques can grow so large that they can block blood flow and reduce the elasticity of the blood vessel, causing coronary artery disease and atherosclerosis. HDLs bind excess cholesterol in the blood and takes it back to the liver where it is broken down, thus reducing the "bad" cholesterol in blood. The other type of fat is triglycerides, which are used to store excess energy from food eaten. High levels

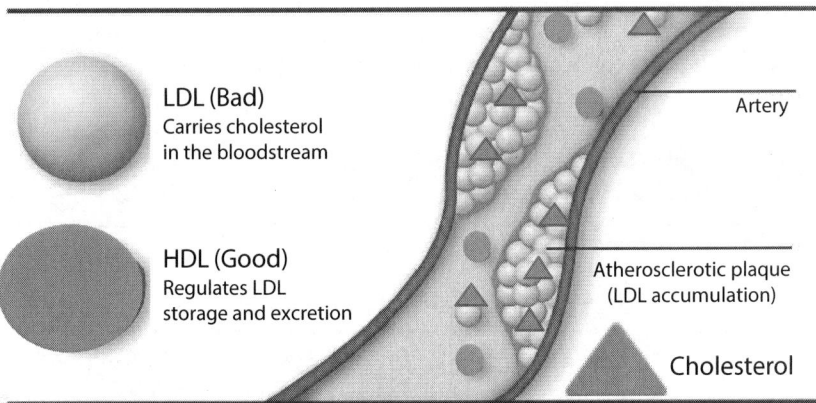

LDL (Bad)
Carries cholesterol in the bloodstream

HDL (Good)
Regulates LDL storage and excretion

Artery

Atherosclerotic plaque (LDL accumulation)

Cholesterol

Figure 4.2 Low-density lipoproteins, high-density lipoproteins and cholesterol. Low-density lipoproteins (LDLs) carry cholesterol in blood vessels throughout the body and deliver it to different organs and tissues. However, if there is excess LDL, then LDL circulates repeatedly in the bloodstream, and will start to build up in the blood vessels by forming plaques that narrow the vessels, eventually causing atherosclerosis. High-density lipoproteins (HDLs) bind excess cholesterol in the blood and reduce cholesterol in the blood vessels. HDL carries cholesterol to the liver, where it is broken down and passes out of the body.

of triglycerides in the blood are also associated with atherosclerosis. Elevated triglycerides can be caused by overweight and obesity, physical inactivity, cigarette smoking, excess alcohol, and/or excess carbohydrate consumption.

Once diagnosed as having metabolic syndrome, a person is at increased risk of cardiovascular disease—in particular heart failure—and diabetes (Alberti et al. 2009). It is estimated that 34% of the adult population in the United States has metabolic syndrome, the risk for which increases with age (Ford et al. 2002). So how can this epidemic in metabolic syndrome be stopped? We do know that attention to good nutrition and increased exercise can help.

It is also important to reduce sodium intake in order to reduce high blood pressure, which contributes to metabolic syndrome. Moderate alcohol consumption, reduced sodium intake but increased potassium uptake, increased physical activity, and a healthy diet in general can reduce blood pressure.

After my breast cancer, I was diagnosed with high blood pressure (no wonder!) and put on a low daily dose of a blood pressure medication. I was so tired of chemicals or any drug in my body, but I knew that high blood pressure is dangerous. So I stopped salting my food, except for a few items that I love with a little salt, and increased my exercise levels. I then noticed that I started getting headaches in the middle of the afternoon. I have never had headaches. Luckily, since I work at a health center, my doctor told me to come to his office the next time I had a headache. I went down to his office and he checked my blood pressure and it was too low. I was taken off my blood pressure medication. Low blood pressure was giving me headaches, and presently I am fine. Now, I only have what I call situational high blood pressure. When I am upset over something at work or home, I can tell that my blood pressure skyrockets, so I am now trying to limit those situations. Otherwise, my blood pressure is normal, especially since I swim three times each week. I do not need that blood pressure medication anymore.

GENETICS, OBESITY, AND HEALTHY DIETS

Genetic research has shown that there are genetic traits that contribute to a person's risk of cardiovascular disease and diabetes. Recent studies have also shown that there is a correlation between genetics and obesity. Various genes have been shown to relate to obesity, and each makes a small contribution to the disease. To solve this issue, scientists combined about 60 SNPs or genetic variants (see Chapter 2 for the definition of SNPs) that are linked to obesity in order to create a panel of genes or a genetic risk score (GRS). Using this GRS, BMI, and the records of the intake of total fat and saturated fatty acid of 2817 U.S. patients, researchers found a significant association between saturated fatty acid intake and obesity (Choquet and Meyre 2011; Casas-Agustench et al. 2014). Although they did not identify a particular gene as being responsible for obesity, they were able to say that limiting saturated fatty acid intake should reduce the fat and BMI of most obese patients.

WEIGHT LOSS

Weight loss programs that result in slow but steady weight reduction (1–2 pounds/week for up to 6 months) appear to be more effective in that the weight loss is able to be maintained, probably due to promoting behavioral changes that stay with the person. It requires that you modify your present diet with small and gradual changes. When you go out and buy expensive packaged meals, it is difficult to eat these meals for the rest of your life in order to maintain your weight, once you have reached your desired weight. However, diet meals do teach people about portion sizes, which are too large in most restaurants than what is considered normal. Reducing the fat in what is eaten now and making other compromises, such as limiting alcohol or sodas, will also help. When burned by the body for energy, fat produces 9 kilocalories (kcal)/g, whereas carbohydrate and protein produce about 4 kcal/g, which produces less energy for the body to make fat. Kilocalories are a unit of measure for energy. A calorie is approximately the amount of energy needed to raise the temperature of 1 kg of water by 1°C. One kilocalorie is equal to 1000 small calories. Thus, limiting fat as well as alcohol (7 kcal/g) is a better way to lose weight. Limiting intake of foods that are rich in saturated fatty acids (e.g., full-fat dairy products, fatty meats, and tropical oils) and trans-unsaturated fatty acids (trans fats) found in prepared foods containing hydrogenated vegetable oils (cookies, crackers, commercially prepared fried foods, and some margarines) can help to keep the heart, blood vessels, and waistline in better shape.

In 2015, the Food and Drug Administration (FDA) determined that artificial trans fat is no longer safe for use in food. Artificial trans fat forms when vegetable oil is hardened by treatment with hydrogen at high temperatures and pressures, converting the vegetable oil into a semi-solid or solid, which occurs in many fast-food restaurants in food preparation. Many foods such as margarine, shortening, and other processed foods contain trans fats. In the early 1990s, clinical studies showed that trans fat might be harmful to health, because it raised the "bad" LDL cholesterol and lowered the "good" HDL cholesterol in the blood. These contribute to stiffening of the arteries and increasing the risk for heart disease and diabetes. Walter Willett (2012) and other epidemiologists at the Harvard School of Public Health estimated trans fats cause approximately 50,000 premature heart attacks each year. This ruling of the FDA is a major victory for public health and was due to a sustained public campaign involving litigation and disclosing trans fats on Nutrition Facts labels. Various cities, counties, and even states had already prohibited the use of partially hydrogenated oils in restaurants.

On the other hand, very-low-fat diets are not recommended unless you are under a physician's supervision. Results of scientific trials show that weight loss on very-low-fat diets is not recommended for three reasons: first, such weight loss is not sustained for many years (Sheppard et al. 1991; Lichtenstein et al. 1998). Second, if someone is extreme with a low-fat diet, then they may develop nutritional inadequacies, especially regarding insufficient fatty acids, which are essential for the body to function. Third, these types of diets are often associated with the use of processed low-fat foods that have lots of calories and chemicals (Rolls and Shide 1992). In addition, we do not know the long-term benefits, safety, and risks of fat-modified products and chemical substitutes for fat.

There is also no solid scientific evidence that high-protein diets result in sustained weight loss or improved health (Krauss et al. 2001). Often, such diets can be very expensive.

EATING HEALTHY

There does not seem to be just one factor in our diet that we can limit in order to lose weight and keep it off, or to improve our health. Rather, it is following a healthy diet for a prolonged period of time that minimizes swings in weight and the chance of obesity. In addition, as we age, we do not need as many calories and we become less active, so our food intake needs to be modified accordingly. However, there are definitely different foods that are helpful or harmful, as we discussed above.

If you read the literature on healthy things to eat, you will find that breakfast is very important. Two breakfast items seem to have great health benefits. First, increasing coffee intake by 8 ounces a day for 4 years reduced the risk of type 2 diabetes by 11% (Bhupathiraju et al. 2014). Interestingly, both caffeinated and decaffeinated coffee produced the same effect (Ding et al. 2014). Thus, it may not be the caffeine, but perhaps antioxidants and other bioactive compounds in caffeinated and decaffeinated coffee that are so beneficial. An antioxidant is a molecule that inhibits the chemical reaction of oxidation involving the loss of electrons, which can create free radicals that start reactions in the body. We do not know all of the reasons for coffee's health benefits, but it is being actively investigated. Second, for those who have cardiovascular disease and/or have had a first heart attack, increasing fiber intake by eating cereal fiber (but not fruit fiber) decreased the risk of death from cardiovascular disease by more than a third (Li et al. 2014).

SUGAR-SWEETENED SODAS

The former mayor of New York City, Michael Bloomberg, banned the sale of extra-large sugar-sweetened sodas in the city. He was criticized severely and praised in the media. There is considerable evidence that greater intake of these beverages is associated with weight gain and obesity in children and adults; even within 12 months, there is observable weight gain (Malik et al. 2006). A large study of patients in Sweden found that consumption of sugary beverages increased the risk of stroke for men and women (Larsson et al. 2014). There is now considerable scientific literature that is too large to cite here on the increased risk of diseases with the overconsumption of sugar-sweetened beverages. If that does not change your ways, maybe the fact that lower semen quality being found in young men who consume large amounts of sweetened sodas will motivate people to reduce their consumption of extra-large sugar-sweetened sodas (Chan et al. 2014).

However, an individual person can be driven crazy by responding to each item that scientists say improves health. The best solution is to have a reasonable, balanced, healthy diet, and then if you are at risk for a particular disease in your family or if you develop a disease, science and doctors can help improve your chances of surviving longer and with fewer health issues by adding, removing, or modifying specific items in your diet.

PHYSICAL ACTIVITY AND EXERCISE

Physical activity is extremely important not only for reducing high blood pressure, weight reduction, or preventing weight gain, but also for cardiovascular fitness and health. Intermittent walking for 30–45 minutes each day of the week and a reduction of sedentary time are recommended.

Too much sitting is detrimental to your health. Humans are not meant to sit most of the day for years on end in their jobs. It is important to get up from the chair every hour. Sedentary behaviors, especially TV watching, have been associated with significantly elevated risks of obesity and type 2 diabetes, whereas even light to moderate activity was associated with a substantially lower risk (Hu 2003). A compilation of many studies on this topic from the same group has shown that excessive TV viewing not only increased the risk of diabetes and obesity, but also increased all types of mortality (Grontved and Hu 2011).

The benefit of walking extends to our mental processes. Walking was shown to increase creativity, and walking outdoors was even more helpful than sitting or being sedentary (Oppezzo and Schwartz 2014). Various tests were given to the students after walking or sitting. These tests were the Guilford's Alternate Uses (GAU) test of creative divergent thinking and the Compound Remote Associates (CRA) test of convergent thinking. For example, students who walked rather than sat were able to think up about 60% more creative uses of an object that were novel and appropriate.

An exciting recent study demonstrates that exercise can cause epigenetic modifications to the DNA (Lindholm et al. 2014). Volunteers were asked to bicycle using only one leg, leaving the other unexercised, which was the control for the study. Only the pedaling leg would show changes related to exercise. For 3 months, volunteers pedaled one-legged, four times a week for 45 minutes. Performance improvements and increases in enzyme activity in the trained leg confirmed that the training response was highly significant. Skeletal muscle biopsies of both legs revealed that the trained leg's muscle cells had differences in DNA methylation (over 800 sites with over 5% changes in methylation) and gene expression, which correlated with each other, and were different from the dormant leg. These changes in gene activity also correlated with the observed health-enhancing benefits associated with increased exercise. Of interest in the future would be to know how long these epigenetic changes last once the exercise regimen is stopped, or if some become permanent.

In conclusion, exercise has many benefits that we are just starting to understand in more depth. Exercise is one of the most important activities that we can do for our bodies, our health, and our medical system.

POVERTY AND CHILD NUTRITION

There are so many topics in nutrition that are crucial for our health and well-being. We have only touched on a few topics.

A very close friend wanted me to touch on the subject of children and nutrition, because he grew up very poor in Connecticut. In fact, often he had hardly anything to eat when he was little. He struggled in school in his early years, often because he was so tired and hungry. He now believes that he might have done much better in school and had fewer social problems if he had eaten three good meals a day instead of one.

The Child Defense Report of 2014 found that child poverty has reached record levels and children of color are disproportionately poor. These statistics are based on the most recent and reliable national and state data "on population, poverty, family structure, family income, health, nutrition, early childhood development, education, child welfare, juvenile justice, and gun violence." What they and others have found is that one in five children—16.1 million children—were poor in 2012. This figure is confirmed by the U.S. Census Bureau's official poverty measure, in which one in five children are living in poverty. Over 40% of children live in extreme poverty, at less than half the poverty level; for a family of four, this means $11,746 per year. Only three other countries in the developed world have a higher poverty rate than the United States: Mexico leads all nations at a rate of 25.79%, Chile at 23.95%, and Turkey at 23.95%. Then comes the United States at 21.63%. It is incredible that such a wealthy nation as the United States has so many very poor people. More than one in nine children lacked access to adequate food in 2012, a rate that is 23% higher than before the recession of 2008. Our wealthy country has a serious child nutrition and poverty problem that we are not adequately dealing with or actively recognizing as a major issue for the success of all our citizens.

Another issue is breast feeding, which is important for all children and especially poor children, because it provides them the best nutrition for the first months and year(s) of their lives. The World Health Organization (WHO 2015) has stated that breast feeding is the most cost-effective, health-providing, and disease-preventing activity that a new mother can do. The American Academy of Pediatrics has also come out in strong support of breast feeding because of so much research showing its significant nutritional, developmental, psychological, environmental, immunological, social, and economic benefits.

It is difficult to stop writing about nutrition, because it is crucial to our personal health and well-being. Nutrition affects every single person in a profound way and is involved in how we develop disease and combat disease. We cannot expect science and our doctors to prevent or cure our diseases without us taking some of the responsibility for ourselves with good nutrition, as well as routine exercise.

REFERENCES

Alberti, KG, RH Eckel, SM Grundy, PZ Zimmet, JI Cleeman, KA Donato, JC Fruchart, WP James, CM Loria, SC Smith Jr., Diabetes Federation Task Force on Epidemiology and Prevention, National Heart, Lung, and Blood Institute, American Heart Association, World Heart Federation, International Atherosclerosis Society, and International Association for the Study of Obesity. 2009. Harmonizing the metabolic syndrome: A joint interim statement of the International Diabetes Federation Task Force on Epidemiology and Prevention; National Heart, Lung, and Blood Institute; American Heart Association; World Heart Federation; International Atherosclerosis Society; and International Association for the Study of Obesity. *Circulation* 120(16):1640–5.

Bhupathiraju, SN, A Pan, JE Manson, WC Willett, RM van Dam, and FB Hu. 2014. Changes in coffee intake and subsequent risk of type 2 diabetes: Three large cohorts of US men and women. *Diabetologia* 57(7):1346–54.

Casas-Agustench, P, DK Arnett, CE Smith et al. 2014. Saturated fat intake modulates the association between an obesity genetic risk score and body mass index in two US populations. *J Acad Nutr Diet* 114(12):1954–66.

Chan, TF, WT Lin, HL Huang, CY Lee, PW Wu, YW Chiu, CC Huang, S Tsai, CL Lin, and CH Lee. 2014. Consumption of sugar-sweetened beverages is associated with components of the metabolic syndrome in adolescents. *Nutrients* 6(5):2088–103.

Choquet, H and D Meyre. 2011. Genetics of obesity: What have we learned? *Curr Genomics* 12(3):169–79.

Deeb, KK, DL Trump, and CS Johnson. 2007. Vitamin D signaling pathways in cancer: Potential for anticancer therapeutics. *Nat Rev Cancer* 7(9):684–700.

Ding, M, SN Bhupathiraju, M Chen, RM van Dam, and FB Hu. 2014. Caffeinated and decaffeinated coffee consumption and risk of type 2 diabetes: A systematic review and a dose–response meta-analysis. *Diabetes Care* 37(2):569–86.

Ford, ES, WH Giles, and WH Dietz. 2002. Prevalence of the metabolic syndrome among US adults: Findings from the third National Health and Nutrition Examination Survey. *JAMA* 287(3):356–9.

Gandini, S, M Boniol, J Haukka, G Byrnes, B Cox, MJ Sneyd, P Mullie, and P Autier. 2011. Meta-analysis of observational studies of serum 25-hydroxyvitamin D levels and colorectal, breast and prostate cancer and colorectal adenoma. *Int J Cancer* 128(6):1414–24.

Grontved, A and FB Hu. 2011. Television viewing and risk of type 2 diabetes, cardiovascular disease, and all-cause mortality: A meta-analysis. *JAMA* 305(23):2448–55.

Holt, PR, N Arber, B Halmos et al. 2002. Colonic epithelial cell proliferation decreases with increasing levels of serum 25-hydroxy vitamin D. *Cancer Epidemiol Biomarkers Prev* 11(1):113–9.

Hu, FB. 2003. Sedentary lifestyle and risk of obesity and type 2 diabetes. *Lipids* 38(2):103–8.

Krauss, RM, RH Eckel, B Howard et al. 2001. Revision 2000: A statement for healthcare professionals from the Nutrition Committee of the American Heart Association. *J Nutr* 131(1):132–46.

Lappe, JM, D Travers-Gustafson, KM Davies, RR Recker, and RP Heaney. 2007. Vitamin D and calcium supplementation reduces cancer risk: Results of a randomized trial. *Am J Clin Nutr* 85(6):1586–91.

Larsson, SC, A Akesson, and A Wolk. 2014. Sweetened beverage consumption is associated with increased risk of stroke in women and men. *J Nutr* 144(6):856–60.

Li, S, A Flint, JK Pai, JP Forman, FB Hu, WC Willett, KM Rexrode, KJ Mukamal, and EB Rimm. 2014. Dietary fiber intake and mortality among survivors of myocardial infarction: Prospective cohort study. *BMJ* 348:g2659.

Lichtenstein, AH, E Kennedy, P Barrier, D Danford, ND Ernst, SM Grundy, GA Leveille, L Van Horn, CL Williams, and SL Booth. 1998. Dietary fat consumption and health. *Nutr Rev* 56(5 Pt 2):S3–19; discussion S19–28.

Lindholm, ME, F Marabita, D Gomez-Cabrero, H Rundqvist, TJ Ekstrom, J Tegner, and CJ Sundberg. 2014. An integrative analysis reveals coordinated reprogramming of the epigenome and the transcriptome in human skeletal muscle after training. *Epigenetics* 9(12):1557–69.

Ma, Y, P Zhang, F Wang, J Yang, Z Liu, H Qin. 2011. Association between vitamin D and risk of colorectal cancer: A systematic review of prospective studies. *J Clin Oncol* 29(28):3775–82.

Malik, VS, MB Schulze, and FB Hu. 2006. Intake of sugar-sweetened beverages and weight gain: A systematic review. *Am J Clin Nutr* 84(2):274–88.

Moreno, J, AV Krishnan, and D Feldman. 2005. Molecular mechanisms mediating the anti-proliferative effects of Vitamin D in prostate cancer. *J Steroid Biochem Mol Biol* 97(1–2):31–6.

Oppezzo, M and DL Schwartz. 2014. Give your ideas some legs: The positive effect of walking on creative thinking. *J Exp Psychol Learn Mem Cogn* 40(4):1142–52.

Park, SY, NJ Ollberding, CG Woolcott, LR Wilkens, BE Henderson, and LN Kolonel. 2013. Fruit and vegetable intakes are associated with lower risk of bladder cancer among women in the Multiethnic Cohort Study. *J Nutr* 143(8):1283–92.

Rolls, BJ and DJ Shide. 1992. The influence of dietary fat on food intake and body weight. *Nutr Rev* 50(10):283–90.

Ross, AC, JE Manson, SA Abrams et al. 2011. The 2011 report on dietary reference intakes for calcium and vitamin D from the Institute of Medicine: What clinicians need to know. *J Clin Endocrinol Metab* 96(1):53–8.

Sheppard, L, AR Kristal, and LH Kushi. 1991. Weight loss in women participating in a randomized trial of low-fat diets. *Am J Clin Nutr* 54(5):821–8.

Thorne, J and MJ Campbell. 2008. The vitamin D receptor in cancer. *Proc Nutr Soc* 67(2):115–27.

Torti, SV and FM Torti. 2013. Iron and cancer: More ore to be mined. *Nat Rev Cancer* 13(5):342–55.

WHO. 2015. Global nutrition targets 2025 breastfeeding policy brief. http://www.who.int/nutrition/publications/globaltargets2025_policybrief_breastfeeding/en/

Willett, WC. 2012. Dietary fats and coronary heart disease. *J Intern Med* 272(1):13–24.

Woolcott, CG, LR Wilkens, AM Nomura, RL Horst, MT Goodman, SP Murphy, BE Henderson, LN Kolonel, and L Le Marchand. 2010. Plasma 25-hydroxyvitamin D levels and the risk of colorectal cancer: The Multiethnic Cohort Study. *Cancer Epidemiol Biomarkers Prev* 19(1):130–4.

5

Other integrative medical treatments

If we are going to personalize medicine, should we not also include some of the integrative/complementary medicine techniques that show considerable scientific and clinical evidence of helping patients and are less invasive with little to no known side effects?

Many Americans are seeking complementary and alternative medicine (CAM) therapies for their personal health and well-being. In the most comprehensive study to date of CAM usage, approximately 40% of the U.S. population used some type of CAM in 2007, with the most common being the use of natural products that were not minerals or vitamins (Barnes et al. 2008). Deep-breathing exercises were the second most prevalent CAM technique. For children, approximately 11% of them had a CAM therapy in that 12-month time period. As discussed in the previous chapter, many CAM therapies are parts of integrative medicine, which includes nutrition and exercise. Natural products and mind–body techniques, such as deep breathing, yoga, and acupuncture, are sought out by patients who cannot or will not use a particular pharmaceutical product for their condition, have a stress-related disease, or cannot ingest painkillers.

Combining allopathic medicine with evidence-based integrative medicine may be helpful to many people. Even if there are no complications known for a particular patient's treatment, personalized medicine may provide a patient with the choice of trying a treatment that is less invasive to their body or that has fewer or no side effects, instead of relying only on pharmaceuticals to normalize a particular facet of their health. For any medical therapy, it is important that the scientific evidence shows that an integrative medicine therapy is effective for a particular medical condition, and not harmful or of no value. Therefore, this chapter will discuss the scientific evidence for some integrative medical therapies in order to assess their benefit for particular conditions and individuals. Only a few integrative medicine therapies, such as acupuncture, some mind–body techniques, yoga, and energy medicine, will be offered as examples.

If four in ten Americans are using integrative medicine therapies, and other countries such as China, Austria, Germany, and South Korea have even more people using integrative medicine therapies (Frass et al. 2012), then why are they so prevalent? One of the reasons is that our society has created excessive stress. New scientific evidence is demonstrating the existence of a complex network of physiological responses encompassing the central and autonomic nervous system (ANS), the endocrine system, the immune system, and the stress system in our bodies. Stress affects all of our physiological processes and leads to disease. Mind–body therapies have been able to alleviate stress for some individuals and promote health. The effects of some CAM therapies on our physiology will be briefly discussed in this chapter. Secondly, integrative medicine appears to promote health and well-being in individuals, otherwise it would not continue to develop and increase in use. Our traditional Western medicine is unable to find solutions for certain diseases, especially chronic diseases; therefore, individuals have sought out CAM therapies in order to alleviate some of their symptoms. Since the attitude of the general population towards integrative medicine is generally positive, the practice of CAM therapies and CAM products has created commercially successful business enterprises throughout the world due to many individuals paying out of pocket. Therefore, monetary factors have also fueled the development of CAM. Finally, journals focused on CAM and integrative medicine, along with recent basic and clinical research, have improved our understanding of the benefits gained from these various modalities.

ACUPUNCTURE

In the United States, the percentage of acupuncture users (past and present) increased from 4.2% to 6.3% of the population—which equal about 8.19 million and 14.01 million—from 2002 to 2007, respectively (Zhang et al. 2012). As more evidence-based studies are performed, acupuncture as a therapy for pain and other conditions will increase even more, according to the National Center for Complementary and Integrative Medicine (NCCIM) at the National Institutes of Health (NIH) in Washington, D.C.

Acupuncture is the practice of inserting and rotating specialized, solid metallic, hair-thin needles (Figure 5.1) into points on the skin that are known as meridian acupuncture points for therapeutic or preventative purposes (Figure 5.2). It is one of the major treatment modalities in Chinese medicine. According to traditional Chinese medicine, the human body has more than 2000 acupuncture points connected via pathways or meridians. These pathways create an energy flow (Qi, pronounced "chee") through the body, which promotes health. Disease causes blockages or disruption of the energy field. Acupuncture corrects these imbalances in the body and improves the flow of Qi. In general, there are few to no major adverse effects of this process, with a few reports of sporadic, slight bleeding or bruising at needle sites (none required medical intervention). Numerous mechanistic studies in Western medicine suggest that the effects of acupuncture are primarily mediated through the neuro-endocrine system (i.e., the nervous system and the glands that release hormones and growth factors) and involving

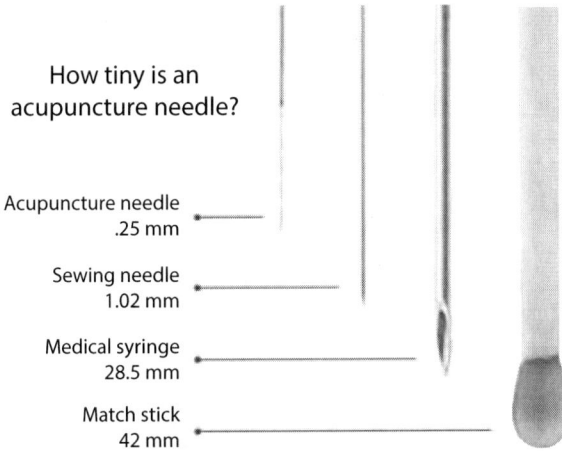

How tiny is an
acupuncture needle?

Acupuncture needle
.25 mm

Sewing needle
1.02 mm

Medical syringe
28.5 mm

Match stick
42 mm

Figure 5.1 Acupuncture needle. The acupuncture needle has a very tiny diameter when it is compared to more commonly known items such as a sewing needle, medical syringe, or matchstick. The acupuncture needle is approximately 0.25 mm in diameter, and so is much thinner than these other items.

the central and peripheral nervous systems with the release of neurotransmitters, including opioid peptides and serotonin in our bodies (Andersson and Lundeberg 1995). However, we still have a lot to learn about the biological basis of the effects of acupuncture.

In a systematic review of well-designed clinical trials, acupuncture appears to be effective for palliative care in cancer patients, especially in reducing chemotherapy, radiotherapy-induced side effects, and cancer pain (Ling et al. 2014). Chemotherapy-induced nausea and vomiting and early postoperative nausea and vomiting in adults are alleviated by acupuncture (Vickers 1996). Acupuncture has also been used to reduce other types of pain, especially from osteoarthritis and other musculoskeletal disorders, as well as dental pain (Ernst and White 1998; Lee 2000). Encouraging but limited evidence has been found for the effectiveness of acupuncture in alleviating acute postoperative pain after back surgery (Cho et al. 2014). Nicotine withdrawal and weight reduction do not appear to be significantly affected by acupuncture (White et al. 2002).

A very close friend of mine was diagnosed with breast cancer: two lesions in one breast. She opted to have a double mastectomy. At that time, she was living alone since her husband had died suddenly 2 years ago. I insisted on taking her to the hospital for the surgery and taking care of her for the first week after the surgery. She had been going to an acupuncturist for routine issues and continued to have acupuncture treatments throughout her cancer treatments of chemotherapy, surgery, and reconstruction. I was amazed at how well she did throughout the whole process; there was very little nausea and vomiting with chemotherapy, minimal swelling, and only a little pain after the surgery. I remember being a basket-case with surgery, chemotherapy, and radiation, and I can only think that acupuncture may have contributed to her ability to handle the ordeal so well.

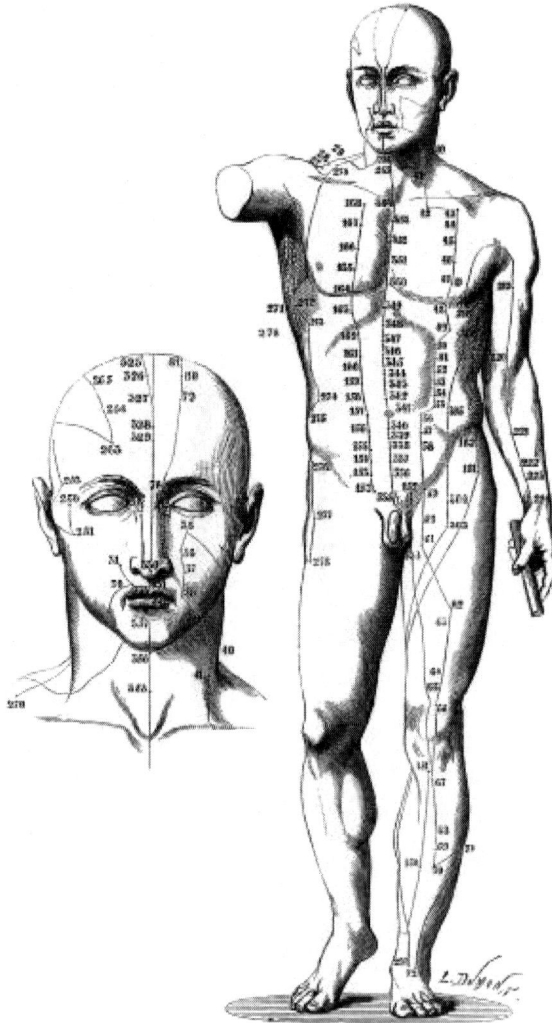

Figure 5.2 A schematic of the Chinese human body meridians (lines running down the picture of a body) and points (numbers) for the application of acupuncture needles. These points affect different organs and aspects of human health. (Courtesy of Wellcome Images, a website operated by the Wellcome Trust, a global charitable foundation based in the United Kingdom.)

With the return of many U.S. veterans from the Afghanistan and Iraq wars, there are numerous soldiers with post-traumatic stress disorder (PTSD) due to their stressful and sometimes catastrophic experiences. Their numbers have been reported to be as much as 6.8%–7.8% for American male veterans and 9.7% for American female veterans (World Health Organization 2004; Olszewski and Varrasse 2005). Approximately 25%–30% of people experiencing a traumatic event later develop PTSD. PTSD is defined by the presence of three types of symptoms in one individual for more than 1 month: re-experiencing, marked avoidance, and hyperarousal. Re-experiencing the original trauma(s) occurs through "flashbacks" or nightmares. Marked avoidance can be seen in emotional numbing or avoidance of the stimuli associated with the trauma. Hyperarousal can be expressed as difficulty falling or staying asleep, anger, and/or hypervigilance. PTSD interferes with a person's ability to cope with their environment and even hold down a job.

The Department of Defense is using acupuncture along with psychotherapies and other approaches, including the mind–body and stress reduction therapies that will be discussed below, in order to help these veterans. It is hoped that these additional patient trials will provide definitive proof of acupuncture's effectiveness in PTSD when these trials are added to the already encouraging data on acupuncture (Kim et al. 2013).

STRESS

Stress is a physiological response to an environmental challenge and can have a positive outcome for the body when the stressor is short lived, but can be detrimental to one's mental and physical well-being if the stressor continues to plague an individual for a long period of time, such as in PTSD. Stress can either be elicited by a physical condition such as confinement or an examination, or can be cognitive, involving mental processes such as upsetting thoughts, memories, or emotions.

The response to stress involves activation of the brain/neural pathways and glands/endocrine pathways with the release of hormones at the same time, followed by changes in the immune system, especially with long-term stress. The neural route for the stress response is quicker and involves the autonomic nervous system (ANS). The ANS controls visceral functions such as heart rate, digestion/swallowing, respiration/breathing, perspiration, salivary secretion, pupillary dilation, urination, and sexual responses. Most of these responses are involuntary or occur below the level of our consciousness in general, but can partner with the somatic nervous system, which allows for voluntary control of some of these functions. The ANS is divided into three subsystems: the parasympathetic nervous system, the sympathetic nervous system, and the enteric nervous system (nerves that govern the gastrointestinal system). These subsystems may operate independently of one other or behave cooperatively. The ANS nuclei in the brainstem receive electrical stress signals from the hypothalamus. The ANS controls the adrenal medulla, causing it to release adrenaline (norepinephrine), which initiates sympathetic nervous system responses, such as increased heart rate, blood pressure, and sweating.

Although a brief description will follow on the body's response to stress, we still do not know enough about how stress affects our physiology, and especially what areas of the brain are affected. In short-term stress, the neural and endocrine pathways work together to produce a maximal response in the body, which is the fight-or-flight response (de Kloet et al. 2006). The physiological changes occurring in the fight-or-flight response give the body increased speed and strength to respond to a stressful or traumatic event. Rapid activation of the sympathetic nervous system leads to the release of noradrenaline/norepinephrine from sympathetic nerve cells, enabling changes in physiology. Some of these changes are increased blood flow to the muscles activated by diverting blood from other parts of the body, such as the stomach, which is not needed in the initial response. For extra speed and strength, muscle tension is also increased. Common changes are elevation of blood pressure and heart rate, along with increased blood sugars and fats in order to supply the body with extra energy. Blood clotting is also increased in order to prevent excessive blood loss in case of an injury.

Hypothalamus–pituitary–adrenal axis and stress

With a stressful stimulus, the cerebral cortex and limbic system of the brain convey the message to the hypothalamus. The hypothalamus can regulate the pituitary gland by a neural or endocrine route. The hypothalamus–pituitary–adrenal (HPA) axis is involved in a slower chemical/endocrine response as follows (Figure 5.3): the endocrine route starts with the secretion of corticotropin-releasing hormone (CRH), which tells the pituitary to release the pre-prohormone antidiuretic hormone (ADH)/vasopressin that was originally synthesized in the hypothalamus, but stored in the posterior pituitary. The pituitary is then stimulated to release adrenocorticotropic hormone (ACTH) from the anterior pituitary. Endorphins are also released from the pituitary and can also be released from the central nervous system. They are naturally occurring morphine-like substances that reduce pain during a stressful experience. Both ADH and CRH help to increase the release of ACTH that acts on the adrenal glands and causes them to secrete corticosteroids, primarily cortisol. Corticosteroids have multiple functions, and they convert fat and protein to useable energy for the stress response. At that moment, nonessential functions such as reproduction, growth, and appetite are inhibited. The effects of the short-term release of corticosteroids is further discussed below.

The physiological events above are also created by the hypothalamus–pituitary–adrenal (HPA) axis, which is comprised of different glands: the hypothalamus, the pituitary gland, and the adrenal glands. The HPA axis also initiates other biochemical pathways in order to deal with stress. The mechanism by which the immune system is recruited is via the activation of the adrenal glands through the HPA axis in order to produce corticosteroids, with cortisol being a major player.

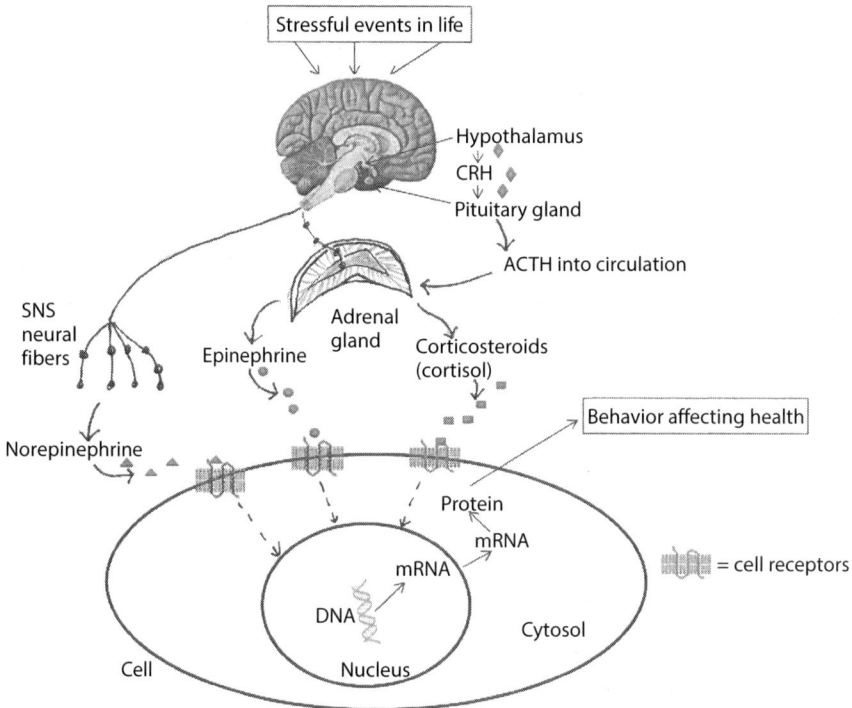

Figure 5.3 Stress-induced signaling pathways leading to changes in health. Stressful stimuli in life affect the brain, leading to changes in the sympathetic nervous system (SNS) and hypothalamic–pituitary–adrenal (HPA) axis. The hypothalamus is involved in the secretion of corticotropin-releasing hormone (CRH), which causes the pituitary to release adrenocorticotropin (ACT) from the anterior pituitary into the circulation. Adrenocorticotropic hormone (ACTH) acts on the adrenal glands, which then secrete corticosteroids, particularly cortisol. With prolonged stress and excessive secretion of cortisol, cells from the immune system become suppressed. Since most cells have corticosteroid receptors, multiple types of cells are affected, including cells of the immune system. Glucocorticoids are corticosteroids, and many genes in cells contain glucocorticoid-response elements, specific DNA sequences that can cause epigenetic changes to genes that eventually affect behavior and health. The neural route for the stress response is quicker and involves the autonomic nervous system (ANS), of which the sympathetic nervous system is a part. The ANS nuclei in the brainstem receive electrical stress signals from the hypothalamus. The ANS controls the adrenal medulla, causing it to release norepinephrine (noradrenaline) and epinephrine (adrenaline), and initiates SNS responses, thereby releasing norepinephrine. Both epinephrine and norepinephrine affect cells/organs, leading to changes in health and behavior (such as heart rate, blood pressure, and sweating). (Modified from Slavich, GM, and SW Cole. 2013. *Clin Psychol Sci* 1(3):331–48.)

Corticosteroids include glucocorticoids such as cortisol and mineralocorticoids such as aldosterone. The adrenal glands sit on top of the kidneys and release hormones in response to stress through cortisol and catecholamines such as adrenaline/epinephrine and noradrenaline/norepinephrine. (The adrenal glands also secrete aldosterone that affects kidney function and androgens that affect sexual features and other processes.) We know that adrenaline increases the activation of the sympathetic nervous system and is associated with energy and excitement in the fight-or-flight response, along with the constriction of small arteries, dilation of veins, and increasing of the heart rate. Cortisol also redistributes glucose for energy to regions of the body that are involved in the fight-or-flight response, such as the muscles. Thus, the central nervous system (brain and spinal cord) also plays a crucial role in the body's stress-related responses. Low levels or physiological levels of cortisol can enhance the immune response and prevent over-responsiveness of the immune system (Jefferies 1991; Wisneski and Anderson 2005). In the bloodstream, cortisol eventually circulates to the pituitary gland and hypothalamus, to which cortisol binds. Cortisol then inhibits the HPA axis so that the body can return to homeostasis in a short-term stress response.

Homeostasis is a property of any system, including the body, in which internal conditions remain stable and relatively constant. An example of homeostasis is the regulation of temperature in a room so that it is most comfortable. In the body, homeostasis is a process that maintains the stability of the body's internal environment in response to changes in external conditions. For example, it is the basis of mammalian life by which mammals maintain a relatively constant internal temperature, unlike reptiles, while the environment is fluctuating in temperature. Homeostasis occurs in many different biochemical processes besides temperature regulation, cell activities, and the organs in the body that are involved in a multitude of activities.

With prolonged stress and excessive secretion of cortisol, the immune system becomes depressed and is no longer in a state of homeostasis. Cortisol is a glucocorticoid. Receptors for glucocorticoids exist throughout the body and on practically every type of immune cell, thus glucocorticoids exert "immunoregulatory" functions. In the cell-mediated or adaptive immune system, there are different types of white blood cells or lymphocytes, such as T lymphocytes (T cells), B lymphocytes (B cells), and natural killer (NK) cells.

Innate immune system and adaptive immunity system

The human immune system consists of two subsystems called the innate immune system and cell-mediated immunity or adaptive immunity system (Figure 5.4). The innate immune system is also found in primitive species and even in invertebrates, and involves phagocytosis, which is the engulfment of materials and microbes, which are single-cell organisms that can invade our bodies. Phagocytosis involves specific factors such as complement, coagulation, and some receptors that are found in physical

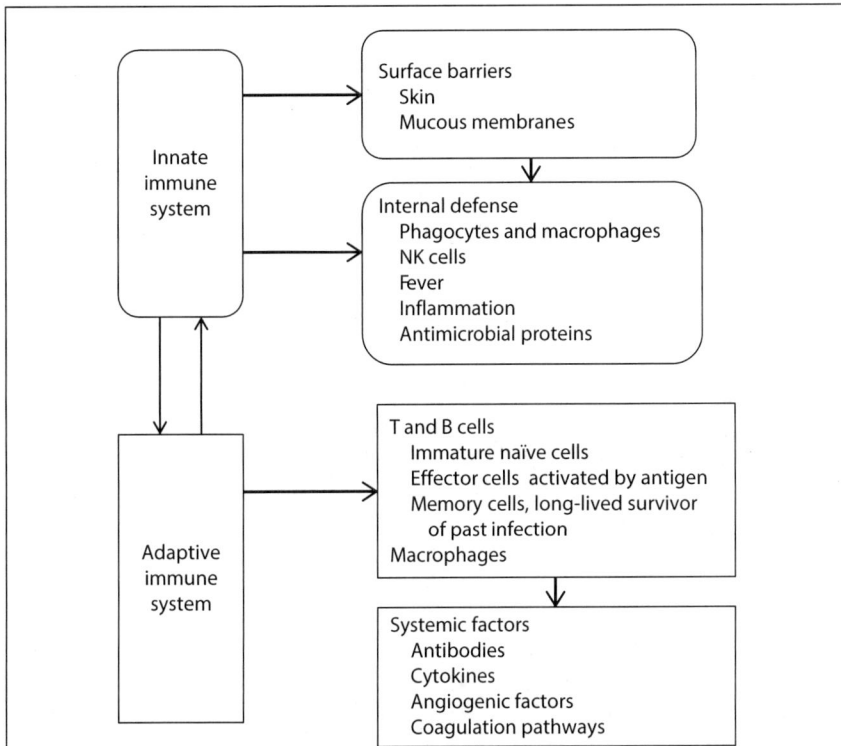

Figure 5.4 Innate and adaptive immune systems. The human immune system consists of two subsystems called the innate immune system and the cell-mediated immunity or adaptive immunity system. The innate immune system involves physical barriers, such as skin and mucous membranes. The cells in the innate immune system are natural killer cells, macrophages, dendritic cells (resident macrophage-like cells in the tissues), and granulocytes (a type of white blood cell). The innate immune system involves phagocytosis or the engulfment of materials and microbes, which are single-cell organisms that can invade our bodies. The adaptive immune system is a more sophisticated defense system marshaling specific cells such as macrophages and T and B lymphocytes. In response to an antigen, they produce angiogenic factors, antibodies, and cytokines, which elicit a more enhanced response with a memory of previous encounters.

barriers such as the skin and mucous membranes. The cells involved in the innate immune system are NK cells, macrophages, dendritic cells (resident macrophage-like cells in the tissues, although they originate from the bone marrow), and granulocytes (a type of white blood cell).

Adaptive immunity is a more sophisticated system in more evolved organisms, and it has the ability to adapt over time and recognize specific pathogens. However, both immune systems interact with each other. This defense system marshals specific cells, such as T and B lymphocytes and macrophages. In response to an antigen, they produce angiogenic factors, antibodies, and cytokines, which elicit a more enhanced response with a memory of previous encounters. Adaptive immunity is also the basis for the success of vaccinations.

Cells from the immune system circulate and recirculate between the central lymphoid organs, such as the thyroid, spleen, and bone marrow, and peripheral lymph organs, such as lymph nodes. The lymphatic system is part of the circulatory system. The circulatory system consists of blood vessels, which process the blood each day. The plasma—the liquid in which the blood cells are found—is filtered in the capillaries. Lymph fluid enters the tissues while leaving blood cells in the capillaries. This lymph returns to the circulatory system, but approximately 10%–20% of the plasma is left in the tissues. It is this lymph that enters the lymphatic vessels, where it is moved by contraction mostly from external tissue forces, such as those generated by muscles. Eventually, the lymph vessels empty into lymphatic ducts, which drain into specific veins (subclavian veins), returning the lymph to blood vessels.

During the circulation and recirculation between the lymphoid tissues, blood vessels, organs, and sites of injury via the blood, cells of the immune system patrol the body by responding to invaders, performing tasks, and developing into more specialized cells.

The blood provides a history of what has happened in the tissues and in the immune system. Sampling the blood provides a "snapshot" of the networks in the immune system, and taking the RNA from a patient's blood can give doctors information on organ-specific autoimmune responses or diseases and whole-body issues. In addition, this approach can present doctors with clues about pathogenesis, as well as potential biomarkers of a disease.

T cells express the T cell receptor, mature in the thymus (although the tonsils can also make some T cells), and become different T cell subsets with different functions. With prolonged stress, cortisol can prevent the proliferation of T cells and inhibit the production of T cell growth factor and interleukin-1 (IL-1), which is a cytokine. IL-1 belongs to a family of 11 cytokines, which are proinflammatory factors that are also able to induce other factors that are important in the response to infections. Therefore, this is one of the pathways by which cortisol suppresses immune function and reduces the production of proinflammatory mediators such as IL-1, as well as other cytokines and chemokines (Bellavance and Rivest 2014). Another glucocorticoid-induced change is the increased differentiation of regulatory T cells that suppress immune function. Glucocorticoids also affect the function and survival of monocytes and macrophages, which clear foreign antigens, pathogens, and cellular debris in the body. Finally, glucocorticoids act on the B cells and affect their function and survival. Thus, glucocorticoids are considered immunoregulators, since they have a multitude of functions that are not always suppressive. Glucocorticoids also cause genomic changes through glucocorticoid-response elements, specific DNA sequences in particular genes to which glucocorticoids bind and thereby change the function of the gene. They can cause non-genomic/epigenetic changes affecting mRNA stabilization and transcription factors that bind to the DNA, among other non-genomic mechanisms (Bellavance and Rivest 2014). All of these changes induced by glucocorticoids profoundly affect the immune system.

Along with the well-recognized effects of glucocorticoids on anti-inflammatory activities, glucocorticoids also affect the brain. Prolonged stress potentiates the expression of proinflammatory mediators in the particular parts of the brain (Bellavance and Rivest 2014). This immune response in the brain was shown to be blocked by RU486, an inhibitor of the glucocorticoid and progesterone receptors (de Pablos et al. 2006; Espinosa-Oliva et al. 2011). Some of the changes elicited in the brain by chronic stress have been shown to cause severe deficits in hippocampus-related memory and increased fear-motivated behavior, which can be attributed to changes in the numbers of specific brain cells, as well as changes in neuropeptides and corticosteroid-induced systems, all resulting in structural remodeling of particular portions of the brain (de Kloet et al. 2006). For some individuals, chronic stress can also lead to depression that can last for months or even years. Thus, a new emerging field of "human social genomics" is developing, in which social–environmental factors and our own perceptions of ourselves can influence the expression of our genes, and thereby protein expression in the immune and neural systems and our ability to combat disease (Slavich and Cole 2013).

STRESS REDUCTION

We have only touched the tip of the iceberg of what chronic stress and anxiety can do to our bodies and our minds. We still have much more to learn. Needless to say, integrative medicine seeks to counteract some of these stress-induced changes in the body and brain. Some of these stress-reducing therapies will be discussed next (Table 5.1). Tai-chi, yoga, acupuncture, qigong, meditation, mindfulness-based stress reduction, and energy medicine are a few examples of such therapies. Some relaxation techniques include autogenic training, biofeedback, deep breathing, guided imagery, progressive relaxation, and self-hypnosis. Then there are adjuvant therapies to help reduce stress, such as aromatherapy, hydrotherapy, massage, music, and relaxation. In addition, very important for stress reduction for many people are exercise programs. Running, basketball, tennis, martial arts, and gym-related activities are some of the exercise regimes that have stress reduction benefits. We do not know which therapy is most effective for stress reduction. Here, too, we have much to learn on particular therapies' physiological effects. In personalized/integrative medicine, we will probably find that individuals respond better to specific therapies that resonate best with that particular person; thus, the personalized approach to stress reduction will be the most effective.

Table 5.1 Examples of stress reduction techniques to promote health and well-being

Breathing exercises that relax an individual

Exercise, such as walking, running, and aerobic exercise. Exercise that promotes progressive relaxation, such as yoga and tai-chi.

Visualization and guided imagery

Meditation

Massage and body work

Biofeedback

Self-hypnosis

Mindfulness programs

Yoga

Energy medicine or human biofield work

Acupuncture

However, it is important to note that in 2008, in a major review of relaxation for the treatment of depression, relaxation techniques were more effective than no treatment for depression, but not as effective as cognitive–behavioral therapy (Jorm et al. 2008) or psychotherapy. Cognitive–behavioral therapy encompasses behavior therapy and mental therapies, and is often "problem focused" and "action focused" for the treatment of a variety of conditions, including mood, anxiety, eating, substance abuse, and tic disorders, etc. We will not be discussing cognitive–behavioral therapies or psychotherapies, which can be very effective for some conditions of depression.

Depression is not always a psychiatric disorder. It can be a normal reaction to particular life events, such as a death in the family, or it can be a side effect of some drugs or medical treatments. Clinical depression that persists for a long period of time needs to be diagnosed by a physician. To be diagnosed with clinical depression, the *Diagnostic and Statistical Manual of Mental Disorders (DSM)*, published by the American Psychiatric Association, is used to determine the relevant criteria, and these criteria are used by mental health providers in order to diagnose and treat mental conditions.

MIND–BODY THERAPIES: MEDITATION, MINDFULNESS, DR. JOHN KABAT-ZINN, AND GUIDED IMAGERY

Since the mind and body are connected based on our physiology as described above, mind–body therapies such as meditation can be helpful in relieving stress and the negative symptoms that can affect the body. In biology, most biochemical processes strive to maintain homeostasis or a steady "normal" state. The environment and internal and other external factors seek to disrupt homeostasis, and if the body strays too far from this state of homeostasis, then an individual experiences stress.

Meditation is a method to self-regulate the mind and is often used to clear the mind of extraneous thoughts and reduce stress. To occupy the mind with less stressful thoughts, some meditation programs recommend a mantra. Mantra is a Sanskrit word (मंत्र) denoting a sound, syllable, word(s), or sacred declaration that is believed to have psychological and spiritual power. There are many different meditation training programs that seek to improve concentration and to promote being in the present moment and not worrying about those things that one cannot change at that point in time or in the past.

A well-known program for stress reduction in the Western world is the mindfulness program, which was created by Dr. John Kabat-Zinn, who is a Professor of Medicine Emeritus at the University of Massachusetts Medical School. The concept of mindfulness has its roots in Buddhism. Dr. Kabat-Zinn developed a Stress Reduction Clinic and Center for Mindfulness in Medicine in 1979. Mindfulness is defined as paying attention to the present moment with a non-judging attitude of acceptance. Meditation is an important part of this program. His stress reduction program has been associated with improvements in health outcomes, particularly for perceptions of pain, anxiety, body image, and reductions in depression, medical symptoms, and pain-related drug utilization (Kabat-Zinn 1982; Kabat-Zinn et al. 1985). His book, *Full Catastrophe Living: How to Cope with Stress, Pain and Illness Using Mindfulness Meditation*, is a classic book in the field of mindfulness (Kabat-Zinn 1990, 2013). Mindfulness practices include body scanning, sitting meditation, and Hatha yoga. Body scanning involves paying attention to one's breath as well as other perceptions in the body while in a state of non-judgmental awareness of other thoughts entering one's head at the same time. These thoughts are then gently pushed aside by returning attention to one's breathing in and out. Hatha yoga involves moving the body through a series of postures to develop strength, flexibility, and body awareness, while still paying attention to one's breath. It seeks to decrease emotional reactivity and lead to a thoughtful and gentle appraisal of oneself.

Another approach to stress reduction is to use guided imagery. Guided imagery involves a program of directing your thoughts or imagination toward a relaxed and focused state. Often an instructor and/or tapes and/or texts are used as ways to help someone relax. Sometimes music is combined with imagery in order to reduce stress.

In a systematic review of mindfulness-based stress reduction articles with strong scientific rigor that combined mindfulness meditation and yoga in an 8-week training program, significant changes in psychological outcomes related to anxiety and/or stress were found (Sharma and Rush 2014). In another review of meditation programs, meditation programs by themselves were shown to significantly reduce psychological stress, including anxiety, depression, and pain (Goyal et al. 2014). However, all authors of these reviews agreed that stronger studies with better controls, experimental designs, and larger numbers of patients would help to define other benefits and the health issues that cannot be alleviated by meditation, so as to provide the best personalized medical approach for a patient.

Leonard A. Wisneski and Lucy Anderson start their book entitled *The Scientific Basis of Integrative Medicine* with the story of Steven, who was a 40-year-old man who appeared in Dr. Wisneski's clinical office for a physical examination. He had a very low hematocrit, which suggested internal bleeding. Upon endoscopic examination, extensive gastric carcinoma was found. Steven was then scheduled for surgery. During his operation, the doctors found that metastasis had already occurred to the lymph nodes and throughout his abdomen, and could not be removed due to the advanced stage of his cancer. In the recovery room, Steven asked his doctor how long he had to live, so Dr. Wisneski replied, "How long do you want?" "Ten years," Steven replied. "You got it," Dr. Wisneski answered. Ten years and six months later, Steven died. His story profoundly influenced Dr. Wisneski's practice of medicine and was the inspiration for his book. In particular, the study of the mind–body connection became a lifelong pursuit of Dr. Wisneski.

YOGA

As discussed previously, yoga was included in the mindfulness program as a method to reduce stress. There is controversy over the historical origin of yoga; however, it is known that the practice originated before Christ and can be found in Hinduism, Buddhism, and Jainism, as well as now in Western culture. Yoga is believed to increase *prana*—or vital energy—in the body and facilitate prana's flow through the body by gentle massaging of the organs by moving the body gently through different positions and improving posture. Although yoga is a physical activity, this ancient practice is considered to connect the mind with the body through gentle stretching, breath control, and meditation. Yoga needs to be practiced regularly in order to receive maximum benefit, but does not require spiritual or religious beliefs.

Yoga has been shown to decrease pain and promote function for a number of musculoskeletal conditions. Yoga significantly decreased lower back pain and functionality compared to usual care (Tilbrook et al. 2011). A number of studies have demonstrated yoga's benefit for low back pain, with some articles demonstrating yoga to be as effective as a program in stretching and better than a usual care program (Sherman et al. 2005). Yoga has been shown to reduce pain intensity (64%), functional disability (77%), and pain medication usage (88%) (Williams et al. 2005), and has an economic benefit due to it being cost effective (Chuang et al. 2012). Other musculoskeletal problems such as carpal tunnel syndrome (Garfinkel et al. 1998) and osteoarthritis (Garfinkel et al. 1994) have also been shown to improve with yoga.

There is also evidence for yoga improving some of the symptoms associated with cancer and its treatment. For breast cancer patients, yoga increased physical functionality, and patients had less fatigue, but there was no significant effect on sleep (Chandwani et al. 2014). For lymphoma patients, another study demonstrated that yoga improved sleep quality (Cohen et al. 2004). A systematic review of cancer patients in different types of yoga programs found promising positive effects on anxiety, depression, and stress, but definitive effectiveness was difficult to assess due to variability across studies and methodological drawbacks of the studies with cancer patients (Smith and Pukall 2009).

In general, many of the yoga studies demonstrate improved functionality and less stress and anxiety with the practice of yoga. In a recent study with students, yoga significantly reduced PTSD and was similar in effectiveness to psychotherapeutic and psychopharmacologic approaches (van der Kolk et al. 2014). A few studies are now starting to appear on how yoga may decrease stress by improving immune function, changing serum cytokine levels (Kiecolt-Glaser et al. 2010), and affecting brain γ-aminobutyric acid levels (Streeter et al. 2010), which may also be some of the mechanisms by which yoga relieves fatigue in cancer patients (Kiecolt-Glaser et al. 2014). However, more scientific work is needed in order to fully understand how yoga can relieve stress and improve immune function.

Energy medicine and human biofield therapies

Although energy medicine or human biofield therapies are a small part of integrative medicine, a recent study on cancer patients demonstrated that these patients reported the highest benefit with energy medicine compared to any other CAM therapies ($p < 0.004$) (Garland et al. 2013). In my own cancer treatments, I tried acupuncture and naturopathic supplements to my diet, and not until I was treated by Therapeutic Touch practitioners, involved in my human biofield studies, did I find that I was able to relax, sleep better, and had less fatigue. Was it just my mind playing tricks on me? Let me show you what I learned about Therapeutic Touch using strict criteria in science.

The concept of a human biofield has its origins in many different cultures over thousands of years with the development of numerous types of biofield therapies—Reiki, external Qi therapy, Healing Touch, Therapeutic Touch, etc.—but only recently has Western science begun to evaluate these practices for their possible therapeutic potential. In this section, Therapeutic Touch was chosen as an example of human biofield therapies because it has one of the strongest histories of clinical trials demonstrating decreased anxiety in various clinical settings (Heidt 1981; Kramer 1990; Gagne and Toye 1994), decreased pain (Keller and Bzdek 1986; Meehan 1993; Peck 1998; McCormack 2009), diminished anxiety and pain (Turner et al. 1998; Lin and Taylor 1999), improved functional ability in patients with arthritis (Gordon et al. 1998; Peck 1998), decreased behavioral symptoms associated with dementia (Woods and Dimond 2002; Woods et al. 2005), enhanced personal well-being in people with cancer (Giasson and Bouchard 1998), and facilitated rest/sleep (Heidt 1981; Cox and Hayes 1997; Cox and Hayes 1998). Many studies were underpowered. However, in a comprehensive systematic review of 66 clinical trials with different types of energy medicine modalities, biofield therapies demonstrated strong and significant evidence for reducing pain and anxiety, as well as having other palliative effects in different clinical settings (Jain and Mills 2010).

Another reason for the choice of Therapeutic Touch as an example of human biofield therapies is the method of practice, which is an uncomplicated, well-defined protocol consisting of four steps that are easily amenable for reproducibility and consistency of practice in a research trial (Monzillo and Gronowicz 2011). The rigorous training program and credentialing process for practitioners—mostly nurses—was also important for consistency in research trials. In addition, there are no religious ties to the practice, so issues such as the role of prayer or religion are not involved in the interpretation of results. Finally, Therapeutic Touch treatments do not require physical contact and can be used in cell culture studies that are sterile.

Personally, Therapeutic Touch has intrigued me since the first experiment in the laboratory in which I tested its effects. My research is in bone biology, osteoporosis, and tissue engineering. Therefore, I was surprised when, one day, a colleague of mine, Dr. Karen Prestwood, with whom I was working on a project on bone aging, approached me with a request:

Gloria, since you have developed well-known methods for growing bone in the laboratory, would you test an energy medicine modality called Therapeutic Touch on your osteoblasts in a culture dish?

She explained to me what Therapeutic Touch was, and told me that she knew of a nurse practitioner who could come to the laboratory to treat osteoblast (bone cell) cultures. I have always enjoyed challenges, so we proceeded.

My technician was away on vacation, and when she returned, I asked her to measure bone formation in the various cell culture dishes without telling her what had been done to them. After a day, I asked her for any results. She replied:

It is very strange, half the experiment worked and the other half did not.

When I looked at her results, I found that Therapeutic Touch treatment twice a week for 10–15 minutes for 2 weeks had increased bone formation three-fold in the normal human osteoblast cultures and had decreased bone formation four-fold in the bone cancer cell dishes. I was amazed, since I had been using the human osteosarcoma dishes (bone cancer) as a model to assess osteoblast responses to biomaterials used in tissue engineering. The normal osteoblasts and osteosarcoma cells had always responded similarly to biomaterials. Here, with Therapeutic Touch, the cells had responded oppositely to each other. I was astounded, and wanted to know if I could repeat these studies. I also had to consider the ramifications of pursuing this work. People might consider me crazy, since human biofield studies are not recognized by mainstream science. However, I also realized that, as a tenured professor, I am supposed to undertake more risky scientific studies, since doing them early in my career would have severely hampered my prospects, whether the results were significant or not. For me, it was the right thing to do, but I made sure that no students would be involved in the project, since we would not be sure of success and acceptance by the scientific community; I would not want to jeopardize a student's career. I also did not become a Therapeutic Touch practitioner during my studies, instead relying mostly on nurses to perform the treatments, so that I remained more objective of my scientific findings.

With these preliminary results, Dr. Prestwood and I approached the National Center for Complementary and Alternative Medicine (NCCAM; now the National Center for Complementary and Integrative Medicine [NCCIM]) in Washington, D.C., to fund our research on the topic. Eventually, I was funded for 5 years, and this work started my research on Therapeutic Touch for more than 10 years. In science, the use of pre-clinical models of cells and animals is helpful in assessing the effect of a therapy and any possible mechanism of action, since one can exclude the psychosocial effects that are found in human studies. Our first studies with Therapeutic Touch were performed on human osteoblast cultures. These studies on normal and bone cancer cells were repeated many times in order to confirm the finding and were published in the *Journal of Orthopaedic Research* (Jhaveri et al. 2008). We have also published our studies with Therapeutic Touch on normal cells (Gronowicz et al. 2008).

Since I am a breast cancer survivor and I have a University of Connecticut Health Center colleague who studies breast cancer in mice, we worked together to determine whether Therapeutic Touch had a significant effect on breast cancer in mice. Therapeutic Touch was shown to have no significant effect on the primary tumor, but produced a significant decrease in metastasis. Analysis of particular cytokines in the sera of the mice and in the immune cells in murine spleen and lymph nodes demonstrated a significant reduction in those cytokines and some immune cell types that were elevated by cancer (Gronowicz et al. 2015). Another colleague has studied ovarian cancer patients undergoing chemotherapy and radiation and has found significant beneficial effects of Healing Touch on the immune system and depressed mood (Lutgendorf et al. 2010).

Biofield research will require many more studies in different laboratories in order to convince the medical profession and other scientists that human biofield therapies have a therapeutic potential. No one knows the mechanism(s) behind the effects of human biofield studies. It appears that these therapies return organisms back to their normal state of dynamic homeostasis or homeodynamics. Energy medicine probably involves electromagnetic fields since our bodies are electromagnetic (for example, our heart can be monitored with electrocardiograms) and probably involves other types of transmittable fields of energy that are fundamental to living organisms that we have yet to study and understand in more detail, but this is very speculative. Is the lack of human touch or human biofield contact partly the reason for the health, behavior, intellect, and emotional development difficulties children face when they spend their early years in orphanages? This is a difficult topic to research, since one cannot control for all of the variables in an orphanage, such as the quality of food, exercise, schooling, and human contact (see http://www.encyclopedia.com/topic/Orphanages.aspx for a history of the literature on this topic).

Does every person have an effect on another person due to a human biofield, and through training could a person intensify these effects? Finally, does this human biofield have positive effects on healing in the doctor–patient relationship, and can these effects be enhanced through the training of doctors?

Why study or use integrative medicine? Diet, exercise, acupuncture, stress-relieving techniques, and other complementary techniques not covered in the last two chapters are, in general, noninvasive, benign (i.e., gentle), mild, and not harmful. Why should they not be prescribed first for what ails us? Why not fund more research on these topics in order to determine their efficacy? Why do we start with drugs, which have many side effects and are expensive, unless it is absolutely necessary? Are we just supporting pharmaceutical companies and their agendas without much regard towards the population at large? Why when we watch television are we inundated with drug advertisement when our doctors should be the ones to advise us on the necessary medications? Let us start with improved diet. Why did I have to be hospitalized while I was on chemotherapy for breast cancer before a dietician came to my hospital bedside? She told me what I should avoid eating, such as a grapefruit every morning, which was my usual routine, but which was intensifying the action of the chemotherapy to my detriment due to extreme side effects. Why, then, did the dietician advise me on what might be helpful to me, such as drinking more water, more numerous smaller meals, and herbal teas in order to lessen some of the side effects?

Let us start with exercise or physical therapy before we resort to surgery. Many orthopedic practices first recommend physical therapy before surgery, and this should be applauded. In the same manner, why not recommend some of the evidence-based integrative methods, such as a change in diet or perhaps adding yoga a few times a week? Why are we not teaching good diet and exercise in public schools, where instead we are cutting these programs, when we know that they will improve health and lessen long-term health cost effects, especially for an American population in which over a third of people are obese? Obesity-related conditions include heart disease, stroke, type 2 diabetes, and certain types of cancer that all burden our annual medical costs of approximately $147 billion. If we are going to personalize medicine, then these non-harmful and noninvasive remedies should be tried first, or at least be part of our doctors' armamentarium for helping us get back to better health. How can any hospital advertise "personalized medicine" without also including complementary/integrative medical therapies?

REFERENCES

Andersson, S and T Lundeberg. 1995. Acupuncture—From empiricism to science: Functional background to acupuncture effects in pain and disease. *Med Hypotheses* 45(3):271–81.

Barnes, PM, B Bloom and RL Nahin. 2008. Complementary and alternative medicine use among adults and children: United States, 2007. *Natl Health Stat Report* (12):1–23.

Bellavance, MA and S Rivest. 2014. The HPA—Immune axis and the immunomodulatory actions of glucocorticoids in the brain. *Front Immunol* 5:136.

Chandwani, KD, G Perkins, HR Nagendra et al. 2014. Randomized, controlled trial of yoga in women with breast cancer undergoing radiotherapy. *J Clin Oncol* 32(10):1058–65.

Cho, YH, CK Kim, KH Heo, MS Lee, IH Ha, DW Son, BK Choi, GS Song, and BC Shin. 2014. Acupuncture for acute postoperative pain after back surgery: A systematic review and meta-analysis of randomized controlled trials. *Pain Pract* 15(3):279–91.

Chuang, LH, MO Soares, H Tilbrook, H Cox, CE Hewitt, J Aplin, A Semlyen, A Trewhela, I Watt, and DJ Torgerson. 2012. A pragmatic multicentered randomized controlled trial of yoga for chronic low back pain: Economic evaluation. *Spine (Phila Pa 1976)* 37(18):1593–601.

Cohen, L, C Warneke, RT Fouladi, MA Rodriguez, and A Chaoul-Reich. 2004. Psychological adjustment and sleep quality in a randomized trial of the effects of a Tibetan yoga intervention in patients with lymphoma. *Cancer* 100(10):2253–60.

Cox, C and J Hayes. 1998. Experiences of administering and receiving therapeutic touch in intensive care. *Complement Ther Nurs Midwifery* 4:128–33.

Cox, CL and JA Hayes. 1997. Reducing anxiety: The employment of therapeutic touch as a nursing intervention. *Complement Ther Nurs Midwifery* 3(6):163–7.

de Kloet, CS, E Vermetten, E Geuze, A Kavelaars, CJ Heijnen, and HG Westenberg. 2006. Assessment of HPA-axis function in posttraumatic stress disorder: Pharmacological and non-pharmacological challenge tests, a review. *J Psychiatr Res* 40(6):550–67.

de Pablos, RM, RF Villaran, S Arguelles, AJ Herrera, JL Venero, A Ayala, J Cano, and A Machado. 2006. Stress increases vulnerability to inflammation in the rat prefrontal cortex. *J Neurosci* 26(21):5709–19.

Ernst, E and AR White. 1998. Acupuncture for back pain: A meta-analysis of randomized controlled trials. *Arch Intern Med* 158(20):2235–41.

Espinosa-Oliva, AM, RM de Pablos, RF Villaran, S Arguelles, JL Venero, A Machado, and J Cano. 2011. Stress is critical for LPS-induced activation of microglia and damage in the rat hippocampus. *Neurobiol Aging* 32(1):85–102.

Frass, M, RP Strassl, H Friehs, M Mullner, M Kundi, and AD Kaye. 2012. Use and acceptance of complementary and alternative medicine among the general population and medical personnel: A systematic review. *Ochsner J* 12(1):45–56.

Gagne, D and RC Toye. 1994. The effects of therapeutic touch and relaxation therapy in reducing anxiety. *Arch Psychiatr Nurs* 8:184–9.

Garfinkel, MS, HR Schumacher, Jr, A Husain, M Levy, and RA Reshetar. 1994. Evaluation of a yoga based regimen for treatment of osteoarthritis of the hands. *J Rheumatol* 21(12):2341–3.

Garfinkel, MS, A Singhal, WA Katz, DA Allan, R Reshetar, and HR Schumacher, Jr. 1998. Yoga-based intervention for carpal tunnel syndrome: A randomized trial. *JAMA* 280(18):1601–3.

Garland, SN, D Valentine, K Desai, S Li, C Langer, T Evans, and JJ Mao. 2013. Complementary and alternative medicine use and benefit finding among cancer patients. *J Altern Complement Med* 19(11):876–81.

Giasson, M and L Bouchard. 1998. Effect of therapeutic touch on the well-being of persons with terminal cancer. *J Holist Nurs* 16:383–99.

Gordon, A, JH Merenstein, F D'Amico, and D Hudgens. 1998. The effects of therapeutic touch on patients with osteoarthritis of the knee. *J Fam Pract* 47:271–7.

Goyal, M, S Singh, EMS Sibinga et al. 2014. *Meditation Programs for Psychological Stress and Well-Being. JAMA Intern Med* 174(3):357–68.

Gronowicz, G, A Jhaveri, L Clarke, M Aronow, and T Smith. 2008. Therapeutic touch stimulates the proliferation of human cells in culture. *J Altern Complement Med* 14(3):233–9.

Gronowicz, G, E Secor, J Flynn, E Jellison, and L Kuhn. 2015. Therapeutic touch has significant effects on mouse breast cancer metastasis and immune responses but not primary tumor size. *Evid Based Complement Altern Med* 2015:926565.

Heidt, P. 1981. Effect of therapeutic touch on anxiety level of hospitalized patients. *Nurs Res* 30:32–7.

Jain, S and PJ Mills. 2010. Biofield therapies: Helpful or full of hype? A best evidence synthesis. *Int J Behav Med* 17:1–16.

Jefferies, WM. 1991. Cortisol and immunity. *Med Hypotheses* 34(3):198–208.

Jhaveri, A, S Walsh, Y Yang, MB McCarthy, and GA Gronowicz. 2008. Therapeutic touch affects DNA synthesis and mineralization of human osteoblasts in culture. *J Orthop Res* 26:1541–8.

Jorm, AF, AJ Morgan, and SE Hetrick. 2008. Relaxation for depression. *Cochrane Database Syst Rev* (4):CD007142.

Kabat-Zinn, J. 1982. An outpatient program in behavioral medicine for chronic pain patients based on the practice of mindfulness meditation: Theoretical considerations and preliminary results. *Gen Hosp Psychiatry* 4(1):33–47.

Kabat-Zinn, J. 1990, 2013. *Full Catastrophe Living: How to Cope with Stress, Pain and Illness Using Mindfulness Meditation*. London: Piatkus, Little, Brown Book Group.

Kabat-Zinn, J, L Lipworth, and R Burney. 1985. The clinical use of mindfulness meditation for the self-regulation of chronic pain. *J Behav Med* 8(2):163–90.

Keller, E and VM Bzdek. 1986. Effects of therapeutic touch on tension headache pain. *Nurs Res* 35:101–6.

Kiecolt-Glaser, JK, JM Bennett, R Andridge, J Peng, CL Shapiro, WB Malarkey, CF Emery, R Layman, EE Mrozek, and R Glaser. 2014. Yoga's impact on inflammation, mood, and fatigue in breast cancer survivors: A randomized controlled trial. *J Clin Oncol* 32(10):1040–9.

Kiecolt-Glaser, JK, L Christian, H Preston, CR Houts, WB Malarkey, CF Emery, and R Glaser. 2010. Stress, inflammation, and yoga practice. *Psychosom Med* 72(2):113–21.

Kim, YD, I Heo, BC Shin, C Crawford, HW Kang, and JH Lim. 2013. Acupuncture for posttraumatic stress disorder: A systematic review of randomized controlled trials and prospective clinical trials. *Evid Based Complement Alternat Med* 2013:615857.

Kramer, NA. 1990. Comparison of therapeutic touch and casual touch in stress reduction of hospitalized children. *Pediatr Nurs* 16:483–5.

Lee, TL 2000. Acupuncture and chronic pain management. *Ann Acad Med Singapore* 29(1):17–21.

Lin, Y-S and A Taylor. 1999. Effects of therapeutic touch in reducing pain and anxiety in an elderly population. *Integr Med* 1:155–61.

Ling, WM, LY Lui, WK So, and K Chan. 2014. Effects of acupuncture and acupressure on cancer-related fatigue: A systematic review. *Oncol Nurs Forum* 41(6):581–92.

Lutgendorf, S, E Mullen-Houser, D Russell et al. 2010. Preservation of immune function in cervical cancer patients during chemoradiation using a novel integrative approach. *Brain Behav Immunity* 24:1231–40.

McCormack, GL. 2009. Using non-contact therapeutic touch to manage post-surgical pain in the elderly. *Occup Ther Int* 16:44–56.

Meehan, TC. 1993. Therapeutic touch and postoperative pain: A Rogerian research study. *Nurs Sci Q* 6:69–78.

Monzillo, E and G Gronowicz. 2011. New insights on therapeutic touch: A discussion of experimental methodology and design that resulted in significant effects on normal human cells and osteosarcoma. *Explore* 7:44–51.

Olszewski, TM and JF Varrasse. 2005. The neurobiology of PTSD: Implications for nurses. *J Psychosoc Nurs Ment Health Serv* 43(6):40–7.

Peck, SD. 1998. The efficacy of therapeutic touch for improving functional ability in elders with degenerative arthritis. *Nurs Sci Q* 11:123–32.

Sharma, M and SE Rush. 2014. Mindfulness-based stress reduction as a stress management intervention for healthy individuals: A systematic review. *J Evid Based Complementart Altern Med* 19(4):271–86.

Sherman, KJ, DC Cherkin, J Erro, DL Miglioretti, and RA Deyo. 2005. Comparing yoga, exercise, and a self-care book for chronic low back pain: A randomized, controlled trial. *Ann Intern Med* 143(12):849–56.

Slavich, GM and SW Cole. 2013. The emerging field of social genomics. *Clin Psychol Sci* 1(3):331–48.

Smith, KB and CF Pukall. 2009. An evidence-based review of yoga as a complementary intervention for patients with cancer. *Psychooncology* 18(5):465–75.

Streeter, CC, TH Whitfield, L Owen et al. 2010. Effects of yoga versus walking on mood, anxiety, and brain GABA levels: A randomized controlled MRS study. *J Altern Complement Med* 16(11):1145–52.

Tilbrook, HE, H Cox, CE Hewitt et al. 2011. Yoga for chronic low back pain: A randomized trial. *Ann Intern Med* 155(9):569–78.

Turner, JG, AJ Clark, DK Gauthier, and M Williams. 1998. The effect of therapeutic touch on pain and anxiety in burn patients. *J Adv Nurs* 28:10–20.

van der Kolk, BA, L Stone, J West, A Rhodes, D Emerson, M Suvak, and J Spinazzola. 2014. Yoga as an adjunctive treatment for posttraumatic stress disorder: A randomized controlled trial. *J Clin Psychiatry* 75(6):e559–65.

Vickers, AJ. 1996. Can acupuncture have specific effects on health? A systematic review of acupuncture antiemesis trials. *J R Soc Med* 89(6):303–11.

White, AR, H Rampes, and E Ernst. 2002. Acupuncture for smoking cessation. *Cochrane Database Syst Rev* (2):CD000009.

Williams, KA, J Petronis, D Smith et al. 2005. Effect of Iyengar yoga therapy for chronic low back pain. *Pain* 115(1–2):107–17.

Wisneski, LA and L Anderson. 2005. *The Scientific Basis of Integrative Medicine.* New York: CRC Press.

Woods, DL, RF Craven, and J Whitney. 2005. The effect of therapeutic touch on behavioral symptoms of persons with dementia. *Altern Ther Health Med* 11:66–74.

Woods, DL and M Dimond. 2002. The effect of therapeutic touch on agitated behavior and cortisol in persons with Alzheimer's disease. *Biol Res Nurs* 4:104–14.

World Health Organization. 2004. The global burden of disease 2004 update. http://www.who.int/healthinfo/global_burden_2004%20update_full.pdf.

Zhang, Y, L Lao, H Chen, and R Ceballos. 2012. Acupuncture use among American adults: What acupuncture practitioners can learn from National Health Interview Survey 2007? *Evid Based Complement Altern Med* 2012:710750.

6

The placebo effect

How will placebo effects change our view of medical treatments?

Human physiology still holds more mysteries that are beginning to be studied, such as the placebo effect. A placebo effect in medicine can be defined as a substance or a procedure that is administered to a person or animal that elicits an effect but does not have any specific pharmacological activity for the condition being treated. As we learn more about the placebo effect, we are coming to realize that it is important for traditional clinical medicine, integrative medicine, and personalized medicine, due to its wide-ranging effects in these areas of medical treatment and the large percentage of people who respond positively to it.

One of the first reports in Western science on the placebo effect was in experiments with rats in 1975. Rats were injected with cyclophosphamide, an immunosuppressive drug, and at the same time were given saccharin-flavored water (Figure 6.1). Later, these same rats were given only the saccharin-flavored water, and the rats continued to display immune suppression (Ader and Cohen 1975). In other words, due to previous conditioning, the rats responded to saccharin-flavored water or placebo as if it were the drug, even though saccharin-flavored water did not have any real effect on the immune system.

We now have considerable evidence of the placebo effect in humans for a multitude of diseases and conditions. Why is this important? Our medical system relies on the results from scientific studies on the effectiveness of pharmaceuticals and procedures to improve health. With positive significant results, these drugs and procedures are approved for use, and they reach us in hospitals, clinics, and at home. If the placebo effect can influence scientific trial outcomes, because some individuals are responding physiologically to the placebo without the medication, then which drugs and surgical procedures are really effective and for which patients and for how long a period of time?

It appears that the placebo effect is part of our normal human physiology and needs to be considered as a component of medical treatment. In randomized clinical trials, the placebo effect was reported to be found in approximately 40% of the patients who have functional disorders such as bowel disorders (Enck and Klosterhalfen 2005). However, fewer than 40% respond well to placebos for other conditions (Enck et al. 2008). Since study of the placebo effects is a relatively

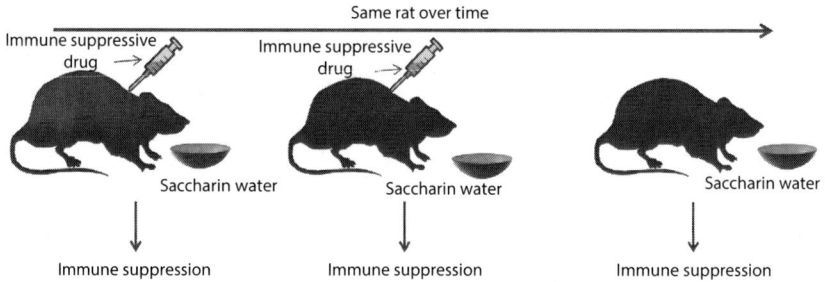

Figure 6.1 Example of the placebo effect. Rats were injected with cyclophosphamide, an immunosuppressive drug, which was given at the same time as saccharin-flavored water for the rats to drink. Later, these same rats were given only the saccharin-flavored water, and the rats exhibited immune suppression. Due to previous conditioning, the rats responded to saccharin-flavored water as if it was the drug. The saccharin-flavored water had become a placebo that elicited a biological response.

young field and irritable bowel syndrome happened to be one of the first diseases to be studied in placebo research, it is not known what other diseases have the same high number of placebo responders.

For much of medicine, placebos have been used as controls in clinical trials, so a particular drug is compared to a placebo pill without the patient knowing which one is which. However, it is required by institutional review boards evaluating the safety of scientific/medical trials at that institution where the clinical trial is occurring—in addition to it being ethical—to explain to patients who enroll in such a clinical trial that they may receive the real drug or the placebo. Many clinical trials use a placebo arm in their clinical trials, and physicians have found that a placebo can elicit positive effects in some of their patients. This can confound the results of the effectiveness of a particular drug being studied. Therefore, it is important to understand the physiological responses that both humans and animals demonstrate in response to a placebo, and tap into this normal response that can perhaps help patients recover from particular pathological symptoms and perhaps even diseases in a less invasive way. There are still many unanswered questions on this topic, such as how long do placebo effects last? For which medical conditions are placebos effective? In which groups of patients does this apply? Placebos are being shown to have powerful dose-dependent effects of their own. An example is a 2008 clinical trial of irritable bowel syndrome in which 62% of the patients had relief from the placebo and their response was dependent on the dose of the placebo (Kaptchuk et al. 2008). Another example can be found in patients suffering from acute migraines. A trial of the drug rizatriptan and a placebo pill demonstrated that both drug and placebo had the same effect (Kam-Hansen et al. 2014).

PSYCHOLOGICAL FACTORS AND NEUROBIOLOGY

The placebo effect seems to involve several psychological factors such as expectancy, the patient–clinician relationship, classical conditioning such as the

Pavlovian response, and anxiety/stress reduction. We do not know whether all of these factors work for each medical condition or if certain diseases and their symptoms are affected in a particular manner during the placebo response. The historic Pavlovian response is now considered as learned conditioning and originated with a Russian doctor, Ivan Petrovich Pavlov, in the early 1900s. Dr. Pavlov started with observations that dogs will salivate before food is put before them in anticipation of eating (Figure 6.2). Then, he discovered that any object, such as a bell or a laboratory assistant whom the dogs had encountered repeatedly prior to feeding, would elicit the same response. We now know that this also happens in humans with all types of conditioned stimuli (in the example above, it was a bell ringing) that, when paired with an unconditioned stimulus (taste of food), will cause the conditioned response (salivation), and this can occur even after only one pairing (Pavlov 1927/1960).

With the study of placebos has come the study of nocebos, which are opposite in effect to placebos. In medicine, a nocebo is defined as a harmless substance that causes a harmful effect in a patient who takes it. Both placebos and nocebos appear to elicit different effects through mechanisms that are dependent on the disease and the experimental conditions, so that a single neurobiological or psychobiological mechanism cannot totally explain all responses to them.

The mechanism underlying the placebo effect is based in neurobiology and has been studied extensively (Enck et al. 2008), but we will only briefly discuss some of its biological basis. The placebo effect has been studied in pain control

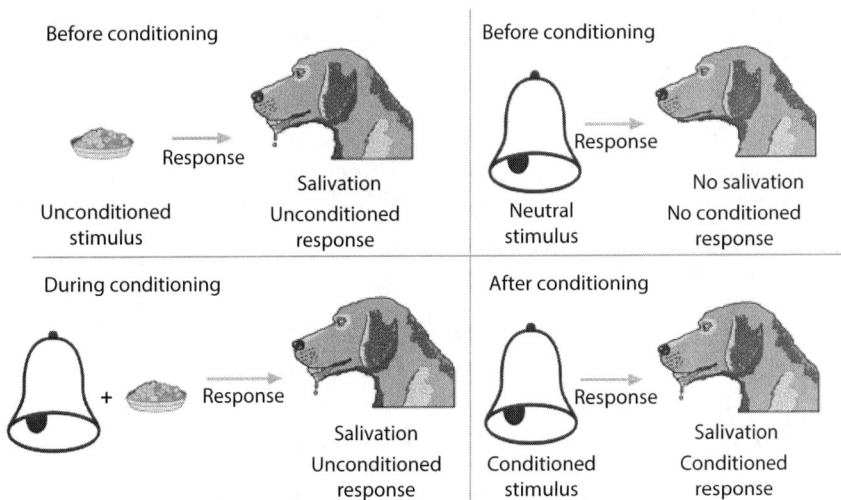

Figure 6.2 Pavlovian response. Dr. Pavlov found that if food is placed before a dog (unconditioned stimulus), then the dog will salivate (unconditioned response) in response to the food. If a bell is rung prior to feeding the dog, then just the bell ringing (conditioned response) with no food being present will cause the dogs to salivate (conditioned response). Thus, the conditioned stimulus (a bell ringing), when paired with an unconditioned stimulus (taste of food), will cause the conditioned response (salivation).

and placebo analgesia, neurological and psychiatric diseases, such as Parkinson's disease and depression, and the above-mentioned irritable bowel syndrome. The placebo effect appears to be dependent on expectation or "brain reward circuitry" (de la Fuente-Fernandez et al. 2002; de la Fuente-Fernandez and Stoessel 2002). The hypothesis is that reward expectations play an important role in the placebo effect. The proposed neurobiological mechanism of the placebo effect is that a positive verbal suggestion is received that may result in a reward, such as feeling better, or in the case of Pavlov's dogs, being fed. In response, particular neurons in the cerebral cortex of the brain, which is the outer layer of the brain, are activated. These neurons send excitatory inputs (using glutamate as the chemical transmitter) to dopaminergic cell bodies (using dopamine as the neurotransmitter), along with indirect inhibitory γ-aminobutyric acid inputs from neurons. These different inputs to the brain contribute to the physiological response. It has been shown that neurons in the prefrontal cortex nucleus, the nucleus accumbens, and the caudate putamen of the brain are activated (Schultz 1998). Scientists can determine which part of the brain is activated by using markers with brain imaging techniques, such as positron emission tomography and functional magnetic resonance imaging. In a study by Scott et al., these techniques were used to show that the placebo effect similarly activated regions of the brain associated with monetary reward (Scott et al. 2007). In addition, the greater someone's response to a monetary reward, the greater was their response to placebo.

Placebo effects have also been shown to activate not only dopaminergic neurons, but also opioid neurotransmission in other regions of the brain (anterior cingulate, orbitofrontal and insular cortices, and amygdala), as well as in the nucleus accumbens (Scott et al. 2008). Conversely, the nocebo response was shown to be associated with a decrease in dopamine and opioid activity in the nucleus accumbens, demonstrating that nocebo responses use the same reward circuits as placebos, but in an opposite manner in order to elicit a negative response.

Other important players in the placebo and nocebo responses in humans are a family of receptors called cholecystokinin (CCK) receptors. Anxiety, feeding, and locomotion are regulated by different CCK receptors through their effects on neurotransmission in the brain. The CCK receptors are involved in the placebo and nocebo responses and can influence such diverse systems as the gastrointestinal tract, pancreas, and central and peripheral nervous systems (reviewed in Enck et al. 2008).

HORMONE AND IMMUNE RESPONSES

Placebo-induced immune responses have also been shown to involve crosstalk between the central nervous system and the immune system. An example of this effect was seen in a series of experiments that were performed under double-blind conditions so that neither the experimenter nor the subject knew whether the drug or saline was being given. Experiments with verbal suggestions to volunteers to release growth hormone and decrease cortisol did not work until subjects were first given a drug (sumatriptan) for 2 days that causes these effects (Figure 6.3). When the drug was taken away and replaced with a placebo,

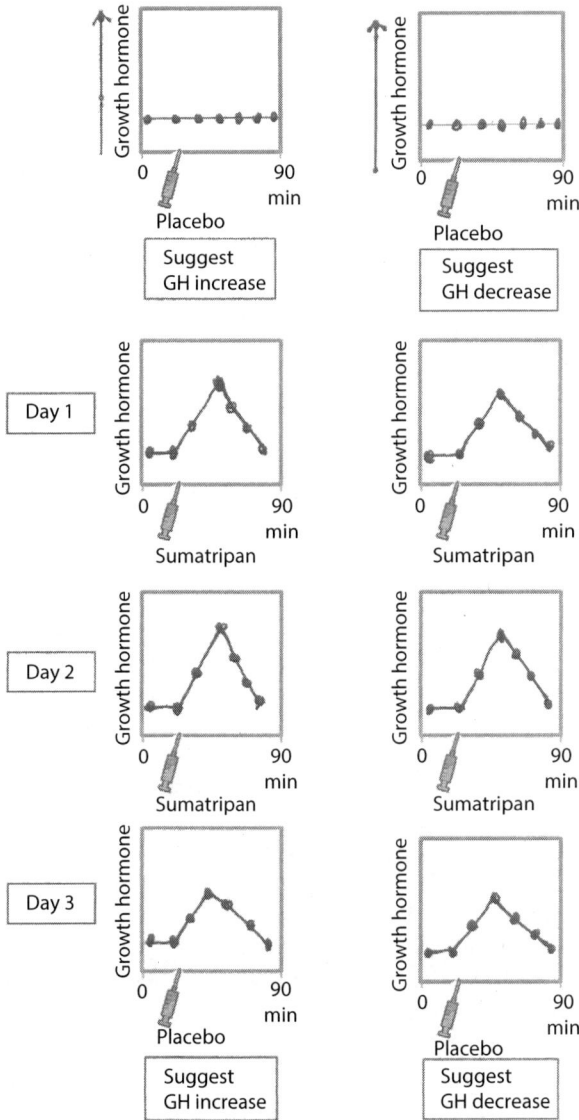

Figure 6.3 Placebo hormone response with conditioning. Verbal suggestions to increase or decrease growth hormone (GH) release (top graphs) had no effect on GH release. If the drug sumatriptan, which increases GH and decreases cortisol, was administered on days 1 and 2, GH levels increased whether the two groups of subjects were told that it would increase or decrease GH. On day 3, the suggestion of GH effects without the drug caused GH levels to increase. Thus, suggestion of GH release is the placebo, and mimics the drug sumatriptan. However, the effect is not caused by the suggestion itself, because the same effect of the drug occurs (an increase in GH) whether the subject is told that it decreases or increases GH. (Adapted from Benedetti, F, et al. 2003. *J Neurosci* 23:4315–23.)

subjects were able to release growth hormone and decrease cortisol release with just a verbal command. If told the opposite verbally (release cortisol and decrease growth hormone), the subjects still gave the same placebo response based on the drug that had previously been given. Thus, the drug was the conditioned response (Benedetti et al. 2003). Experimental evidence has shown that allergic responses or hormone releases that respond to a placebo are due to behavioral conditioning, since they are unconscious physiological responses, while conscious physiological pain and motor mechanisms that respond to a placebo are due to a patient's expectations (Enck et al. 2008).

PLACEBO AND ANTIDEPRESSANTS

Nowhere has the response to a placebo been as controversial as in antidepressant studies. Scientists and physicians are now reanalyzing the benefits and issues with antidepressant medications, evaluating the physiological and biological bases behind the placebo response, and re-evaluating the benefits of physician–patient interactions. A recent series of meta-analyses of randomized clinical trials failed to find significant differences in effectiveness between a placebo and a drug considered to be effective for varying degrees of depression from mild to severe (Kirsch et al. 2008; Turner et al. 2008; Fournier et al. 2010). Meta-analyses are well-accepted statistical methods for combining and contrasting different published studies in order to identify the statistical significance of particular treatments, or to identify particular differences or patterns of agreement between multiple studies.

A number of studies from different clinical practices and laboratories have confirmed the effects of a placebo on patients with depression. When the side effects from these psychotropic drugs are considered, it is difficult to recommend that a patient should take a drug for depression for life. Yet many of these patients have difficulty functioning in everyday activities, and in some rare cases, no treatment leads to harm to the patients themselves or, rarest of all, to other people. Perhaps the most eloquent assessment of these issues and the placebo effect comes from the conclusions of a recent published meta-analysis of treatments and depression from Khan et al. (2012): "In conclusion, the combination of psychotherapy and antidepressants for depression may provide a slight advantage whereas antidepressants alone and psychotherapy alone are not significantly different from alternative therapies or active intervention controls. These data suggest that type of treatment offered is less important than getting depressed patients involved in an active therapeutic program. Future research should consider whether certain patient profiles might justify a specific treatment modality." (Some alternative therapies in the literature that Khan et al. referenced were acupuncture, exercise, and relaxation protocols, while active intervention controls were sham acupuncture and therapies not specific to depression.) This study also cautioned that those individuals with depression who enroll in a scientific study may differ from those who do not, so the results may not be universally applicable. A recent meta-analysis of antidepressants versus placebo found increased overall well-being and decreased depression symptoms with placebo treatment of young people (Spielmans and Gerwig 2014). Therefore, the placebo effect has even been found in children and young adults.

PLACEBO EFFECT, SURVIVAL EFFECTS, AND OTHER QUESTIONS

As can be seen from the few examples given on placebo studies, this field of study is very controversial but very important for our individualized medical care. One additional interesting finding that has arisen from placebo response trials is that patients that adhere to medication instructions for greater than 80% of the time have a better survival from coronary artery disease (The Coronary Drug Project Research Group 1980). Those patients with poor drug adherence had a higher risk of myocardial infarction and mortality (Horwitz et al. 1990). In both studies, the survival effects were similar whether the patients were given a placebo or the active compound. Placebo effects involve not only the ingestion of a sugar pill, but also include patient–doctor interactions, trust, compassion, the patient's medical beliefs, and the ritual in the therapeutic experience.

Other interesting questions that have arisen from placebo studies are: how long can a placebo effect be maintained? Are all diseases and symptoms susceptible to placebo effects? How has the placebo effect influenced the development and validation of new medical treatments in clinical trials? Which individuals are particularly responsive to placebos and which to nocebos? Obviously, additional scientific studies need to be performed in order to answer these questions; however, the power of behavioral conditioning and our expectations in our responses to medical treatments cannot be minimized. In addition, the placebo effect has the potential to enhance medical treatments and to provide therapeutic benefits on its own. However, care must be taken with the analysis of placebo effects so as not to discourage pharmaceutical therapies for patients who do not respond to a placebo and need their medications for their health and well-being.

REFERENCES

Ader, R and N Cohen. 1975. Behaviorally conditioned immunosuppression. *Psychosom Med* 37(4):333–40.

Benedetti, F, A Pollo, L Lopiano, M Lanotte, S Vighetti, and M Rainero. 2003. Conscious expectation and unconscious conditioning in analgesis, motor, and hormonal placebo/nocebo responses. *J Neurosci* 23:4315–4323.

de la Fuente-Fernandez, R, M Schulzer, and AJ Stoessel. 2002. The placebo effect in neurological disorders. *Lancet Neurol* 1:85–91.

de la Fuente-Fernandez, R and AJ Stoessel. 2002. The placebo effect in Parkinson's disease. *Trends Neurosci* 25:302–306.

Enck, P, F Benedetti, and M Schedlowski. 2008. New insights into the placebo and nocebo responses. *Neuron* 59:195–206.

Enck, P and S Klosterhalfen. 2005. The placebo response in functional bowel disorders: Perspectives and putative mechanisms. *Neurogastroenterol Motil* 17:325–331.

Fournier, JC, RJ DeRubeis, SD Hollon, S Dimidjian, JD Amsterdam, RC Shelton, and J Fawcett. 2010. Antidepressant drug effects and depression severity. *JAMA* 303(1):47–53.

Horwitz, RI, CM Viscoli, L Berkman, RM Donaldson, SM Horwitz, CJ Murray, DF Ransohoff, and J Sindelar. 1990. Treatment adherence and risk of death after a myocardial infarction. *Lancet* 336:542–545.

Kam-Hansen, S, M Jakubowski, JM Kelley, I Kirsch, DC Hoaglin, TJ Kaptchuk, and R Burstein. 2014. Altered placebo and drug labeling changes the outcome of episodic migraine attacks. *Sci Transl Med* 6(218):218ra5.

Kaptchuk, TJ, JM Kelley, LA Conboy et al. 2008. Components of placebo effect: Randomised controlled trial in patients with irritable bowel syndrome. *BMJ* 336(7651):999–1003.

Khan, A, J Faucett, P Lichtenberg, I Kirsch, and WA Brown. 2012. A systematic review of comparative efficacy of treatments and controls for depression. *PLoS One* 7(7):e41778.

Kirsch, I, BJ Deacon, TB Huedo-Medina, A Scoboria, TJ Moore, and BT Johnson. 2008. Initial severity and antidepressant benefits: A meta-analysis of data submitted to the Food and Drug Administration. *PLoS One* 5(2):e45.

Pavlov, IP. 1927/1960. *Conditioned Reflexes: An Investigation of the Physiological Activity of the Cerebral Cortex*. Translated and edited by GV Anrep. London: Oxford University Press.

Schultz, W. 1998. Predictive reward signal of dopamine neurons. *J Neurophysiol* 80:1–27.

Scott, DJ, CS Stohler, CM Egnatuk, H Wang, RA Koeppe, and JK Zubieta. 2007. Individual differences in reward responding explain placebo-induced expectations and effects. *Neuron* 55(2):325–36.

Scott, DJ, CS Stohler, CM Egnatuk, H Wang, RA Koeppe, and JK Zubieta. 2008. Placebo and nocebo effects are defined by opposite opioid and dopaminergic responses. *Arch Gen Psychiatry* 65:220–231.

Spielmans, GI and K Gerwig. 2014. The efficacy of antidepressants on overall well-being and self-reported depression symptom severity in youth: A meta-analysis. *Psychother Psychom* 83:158–164.

The Coronary Drug Project Research Group. 1980. Influence of adherence to treatment and response of cholesterol on mortality in the coronary drug project. *N Engl J Med* 303:1038–1041.

Turner, EH, AM Mathews, E Linardatos, RA Tell, and R Rosenthal. 2008. Selective publication of antidepressant trials and its influence on apparent efficacy. *N Engl J Med* 358:252–260.

7

Stem cells

Stem cell biology is a powerful tool, but is it ready to be applied to medical conditions?

The bionic man and woman of the 1970s may become a reality in the twenty-first century. However, the replacement parts would originate from your own tissues through stem cell biology, or that is the hope.

STEM CELLS IN MEDICINE

As human lifespan increases, medicine is dealing with the increased need to regenerate organs or tissues for older patients or for when organs fail due to intractable diseases such as renal failure, liver cirrhosis, Alzheimer's and Parkinson's disease, or simply aging. Renal and liver transplantation have helped numerous patients. However, the shortage of immune-matched organs, and issues with them such as serious infections due to immunosuppression from the drugs that are necessary for organ acceptance, have hampered transplantation medicine. Advances in stem cell research have given new promise for personalizing cell or organ therapies for human diseases (Robinton and Daley 2012; Papp and Plath 2013). Stem cells are unspecialized cells found in most tissues that have the ability to renew themselves or remain dormant until they are needed to regenerate a tissue on a limited basis in animals and in humans. We can observe the capability of this remarkable process in some amphibians such as salamanders and newts that have the ability to regenerate tails, limbs, and even eyes.

EMBRYONIC STEM CELLS

Unlike salamanders, human adult stem cells are limited in their regeneration depending on the tissue. Scientists have devised other approaches using stem cells derived from embryos to generate new tissues. Embryonic stem cells (ESCs) were discovered in 1981 by Evans and Kaufman (1981) and Martin (1981). In early human development, the oocyte, once activated in fertilization by a sperm, has the capacity for a limited amount of time in development to produce all of the tissues in a mature organism. ESCs are derived from the inner cell mass of the blastocyst, an early embryonic stage in development, and consist of cells that

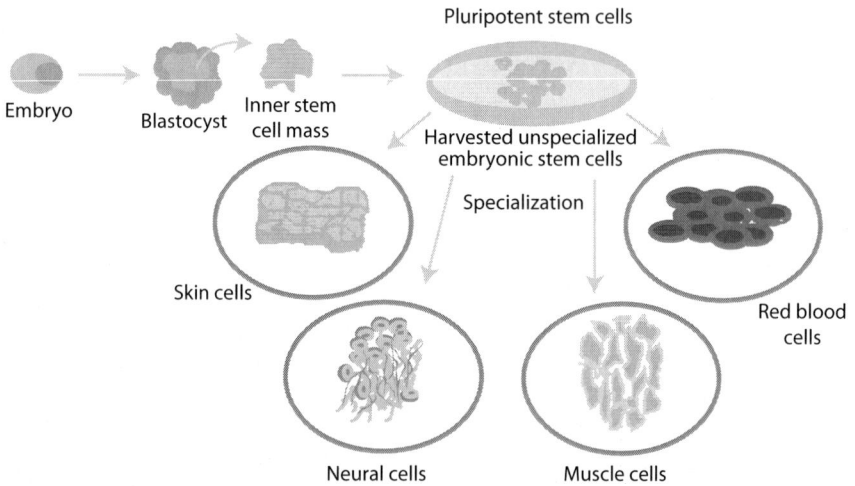

Figure 7.1 Embryonic stem cells. Embryonic stem cells are derived from embryos that have reached the blastocyst stage of 3–5 days old and are hollow balls. The inner cell mass of the blastocyst is placed in the culture dish with a feeder layer (often mouse skin cells) and cell culture medium necessary for their growth. After days of growth, only the stem cells are plated onto new culture dishes, upon which they are grown for months as unspecialized cells. Then, different dishes of these cells can be fed with different types of media, specific for a particular cell type, which will allow them to differentiate in order to become either skin cells or neural cells, etc. (Adapted from *Structural Biochemistry/Stem Cells*, Wikibooks.)

are capable of making any tissue type (i.e., they are pluripotent) (Figure 7.1). A pluripotent cell is defined as a cell that can generate cell types from each of the three embryonic germ cell layers: endoderm, mesoderm, and ectoderm. ESCs at this early stage in human development can be used in the laboratory to generate new tissues (Figure 7.1). As the embryo matures with age, this potential is lost.

The use of cells from embryos for medical experimentation had a pitfall. The destruction of human embryos for science had moral and ethical ramifications, and became very controversial. In addition, in vitro fertilization was developed and involved a process of fertilization in which an egg and sperm are manually combined in a laboratory dish, and then this embryo is transferred to a woman's uterus for continued development into a normal baby.

The first successful in vitro fertilization procedure leading to a birth occurred in 1978. In response to these new scientific advances, the federal government created regulations barring the use of federal funds for any experimentation on human embryos. This regulation was modified due to the National Institutes of Health (NIH) Human Embryo Research Panel recommending federal funding for research using embryos solely for scientific research. The Clinton administration would not go along with this recommendation. Instead, the administration wanted to fund research for tissue engineering on leftover embryos from in vitro fertility programs. Congress disagreed even more and intervened with the Dickey Amendment in 1995, which President Clinton signed into law, prohibiting any federal funding for the Department of Health and Human Services (HSS) for research that resulted in the destruction of any human embryo, regardless of the source.

Finally, in 2001, President Bush allowed federal funds to be used to fund research that used existing human ESC lines, but not research that would result in the destruction of a human embryo, even to make a new cell line. In the past, neither Congress nor any president ever prohibited private funding of embryonic research. In 2009, President Obama allowed federal research funds for the use of new stem cell lines that were created with private or state-level funds, and this new provision was called The Omnibus Appropriations Act of 2009. However, at this point in time, the limited number of stem cell lines approved for research had hindered scientific advancement due to the small number of cell lines lacking the diversity to answer all of the questions generated with regards to their use as disease models or for treating specific diseases.

INDUCED PLURIPOTENT STEM CELLS

In response to the controversy over ESCs, Shinya Yamanaka and his colleagues in 2006 developed murine induced pluripotent stem cells (iPSCs) (Takahashi and Yamanaka 2006) and then human iPSCs in 2007 from adult human cells (Takahashi et al. 2007). He showed that the introduction of four specific transcription factors could convert an adult stem cell with limited abilities to generate all tissues and complete organs into a pluripotent stem cell that would have this capacity (Figure 7.2). He was awarded the Nobel Prize in 2012 along with Sir John Gurdon, who pioneered nuclear transfer, an important technique for reprogramming cells in order to make a new tissue (Figure 7.3). The advantage of using iPSCs instead of ESCs is that the immune system will not reject iPSCs if they are created by using a patient's own cells for transplantation.

Immune rejection occurs due to the activity of T lymphocytes or T cells, a type of white blood cell in the circulation/body that has a central role in cell-mediated immunity. They are called T cells due to the presence of a T cell receptor on the cell surface that distinguishes the T cells from other lymphocytes, such as B cells and natural killer cells. Most T cells mature in the thymus, although some also mature in the tonsils; therefore, they are called T cells. There are many different types of subsets of T cells with different functions in immune responses. Immune rejection leads to acute rejection or chronic rejection of the transplanted tissue or cells. In chronic rejection, the transplanted tissue can be replaced by fibrotic tissue, which is excess fibrous connective tissue, similar to scar tissue.

iPSCs AND YAMANAKA FACTORS

The iPSCs are created by introducing a specific group of pluripotent genes or reprogramming factors into a cell. The original reprogramming factors, also called Yamanaka factors, were the genes OCT4 (also known as Pou5f1), SOX2, cMYC, and Kruppel-like factor 4 (KLF4) (Figure 7.2). Although these factors

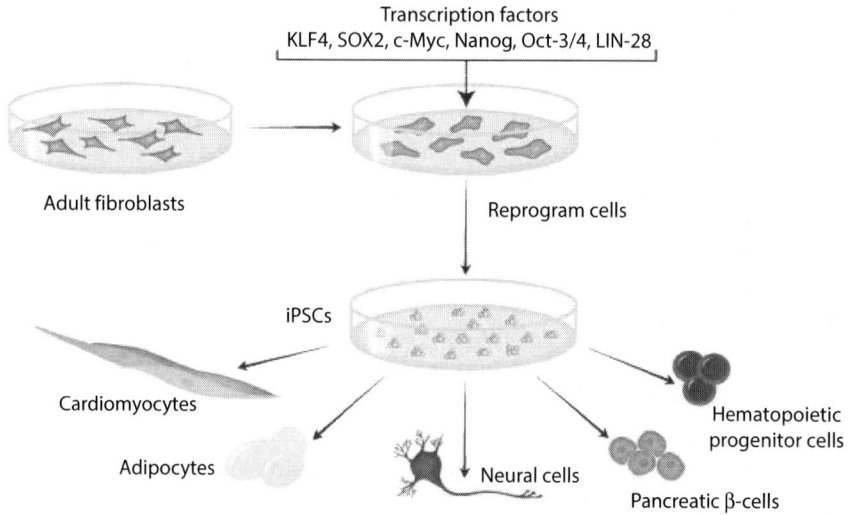

Figure 7.2 Formation of induced pluripotent stem cells. Induced pluripotent stem cells (iPSCs) are created by reprogramming adult somatic cells, such as fibroblasts. Somatic cells are isolated from a person and then transduced with various vectors encoding transcription factors, which allow the adult cells to become pluripotent. For most cells, the transcription factors c-Myc, Oct-3/4, SOX2, and KLF4 are used, but other alternative factors can be used. These transcription factors silence markers of differentiation for the adult cells and induce pluripotent markers, thus reprogramming the cells into iPSCs that have the ability to generate all cell types in the body, such as cardiomyocytes, adipocytes, neural cells, pancreatic β-cells, and hematopoietic cells, etc. (Adapted from Amabile, G, and A Meissner. 2009. *Trends Mol Med* 15:59–68.)

are most typically used, each one can now be replaced with related transcription factors, miRNAs, or other small molecules and even genes that determine cell lineage. This discovery led to the reprogramming of human fibroblasts (Takahashi et al. 2007; Yu et al. 2007; Park et al. 2008). Both iPSCs and ESCs are pluripotent and thus can give rise to a complete organism with every cell type.

SOMATIC CELL NUCLEAR TRANSFER

The technology for creating iPSCs is rooted in somatic cell nuclear transfer (SCNT) (Figure 7.3). In all mammals, including humans, the genes are the same in all cells regardless of the differentiation or expression of a particular set of proteins that make up that particular tissue. If one removes the nucleus from a fertilized egg and then transfers by SCNT an adult nucleus into this enucleated egg, then that nucleus is reset to develop once again into a cell as determined by the donor nucleus (Briggs and King 1952). Cloning is the process of producing similar populations of genetically identical individuals. In 1962, Gurdon was the first to successfully clone an organism, which was a frog, *Xenopus*. Tadpole intestinal or muscle cells were transferred into enucleated *Xenopus* eggs, which gave

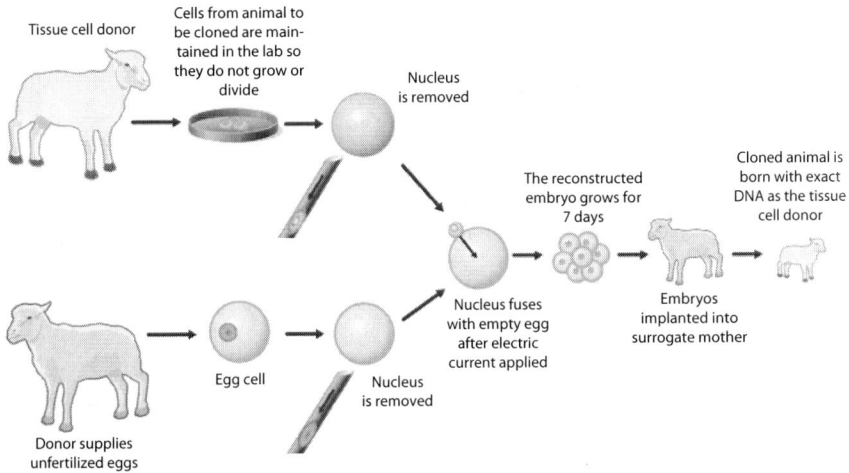

Figure 7.3 Somatic nuclear transfer. This technique involves the removal of the nucleus from a fertilized egg—creating an enucleated egg—and then transferring an adult donor nucleus into that enucleated egg. The nucleus is reset to develop once again into a cell determined by the donor nucleus. The first cloning of a mammal was a sheep named Dolly. (Data from http://cloningdc. weebly.com/technology.html. Accessed on March 6, 2016.)

rise to complete, mature frogs (Gurdon 1962). The first cloning of a mammal was of a sheep named Dolly. One of the promises of this technology is that eventually researchers would be able to create pluripotent stem cells specific to each patient for personalized medicine. One of the pitfalls of this technology is the concern that human beings could theoretically be cloned. Another pitfall is that we still do not know whether iPSCs created from an aged person's nucleus or other aged animal's nucleus differentiate normally (Isobe et al. 2014). There appears to be premature aging in some cases, due to multiple factors in the cell that are different from ESC-derived cells and organisms.

SCIENTIFIC PROBLEMS TO BE SOLVED FOR iPSCs

Before we can clinically apply iPSC methodologies, a number of potential problems must be solved (Table 7.1). When cells are reprogrammed in order to create a new organism, DNA mutations, duplications, and rearrangements are more prevalent and can cause abnormal development. Scientists still do not know whether these changes in the DNA occur due solely to the scientific procedure in reprogramming, or also due to variations that already existed in the tissue that was used to create the iPSCs (Mayshar et al. 2010; Laurent et al. 2011).

Examples of how scientific procedures may affect gene expression are as follows: first, chromosomal aberrations are common in stem cell populations that have been propagated in vitro, whether they are iPSCs or ESCs. The more that cells are passaged in a laboratory in order to expand the number of

Table 7.1 Advantages and disadvantages of using induced pluripotent stem cells (iPSCs) for tissue engineering

Advantages of iPSCs

Derived from adult patients in order to study the cellular basis of a patient's disease

Since iPSCs are self-renewing and pluripotent, they represent a theoretically unlimited source of patient-derived cells, which can be turned into any type of cell in the body

Collection of iPSC lines for drug screening for a particular disease

Useful for disease modeling

Generate human organs for transplantation

Tissue repair using stem cells engrafted into the injured or diseased tissue

Create Type O blood cells that can be transfused into all patients

Disadvantages of iPSCs

DNA changes: mutations, rearrangements, and duplications

Cell function affected by the use of gene insertions using retroviruses or oncogenes

Epigenetic variations between iPSCs; degree of methylation

Teratoma formation

Immunogenicity even in syngenetics, leading to immune rejection

Memory of past cell identity retained by iPSC

Oncogene expression: all of the genes that have been shown to promote iPSC formation have also been linked to cancer in one way or another, and some of the genes are known oncogenes

Some solutions

Develop non-genetic methods of producing iPSCs using recombinant proteins, and improve their efficiency, creating safer iPSCs

Set up rules for cell passaging and limit cell passage numbers

---

cells for scientific study, the more chromosomal changes occur; for example, chromosome copy numbers start to vary. Second, scientific procedures, such as using retroviruses or oncogenes to insert new genes for a particular type of cell development or cell phenotype, can affect cell function. In addition, we know that transcriptional and epigenetic variations are common between ESC lines and iPSC lines (Kim et al. 2010), and we do not know all of the reasons as to why this is the case. Epigenetic differences between iPSCs and ESCs—in particular in the degree of methylation (i.e., suppression of particular genes)—have been found. It is not known how these varying epigenetic differences will alter the differentiation potential of iPSCs (Robinton and Daley 2012). Will all of the tissue be functionally normal, or will there be problems as the tissue develops?

Another issue that needs study is the formation of teratomas or other tumors with the use of iPSC and ESC technologies (Gropp et al. 2012; Isobe et al. 2014).

Teratomas are benign tumors that form multiple types of tissues; even hair and eyes have been found in teratomas. Although a teratoma is benign, it can grow very large, and then cause health problems and even death. In addition, when teratocarcinomas occur from iPSC technology, they are more aggressive than the teratocarcinomas that develop from human ESCs (hESCs). Finally, there are issues of immunogenicity in syngeneic recipients (i.e., iPSCs transplanted from a patient's own cells or even from a mouse's own cells into that same mouse) (Zhao et al. 2011). Immune rejection can occur, and we do not know all of the reasons why and in which situations this occurs. In general, the scientific data suggest that the differentiation potential of an iPSC is influenced by its parental origin. In other words, an iPSC may retain a "memory" of its past identity as a particular cell type, which may cause some of the problems with iPSCs (Robinton and Daley 2012).

In order to solve many of these problems in the future, it will be important to develop a consensus among scientists as to the most consistent and optimal protocols for creating iPSCs (Table 7.1). More rigorous controls to ensure consistency between laboratories are needed. It is also critical to minimize the time of cells in culture and define the best protocol for cell culture at all stages. In spite of the need for further research, the NIH closed their Center for Regenerative Medicine and stem cell program in 2014, after awarding only one grant to Dr. Bharti of the National Eye Institute of the NIH. Dr. Bharti will use iPSC-derived retinal pigment epithelium (RPE) cells to improve the sight of patients with macular degeneration. The RPE cell is the cell that is damaged in macular degeneration. Additional funding and a new process for funding stem cell research should be developed soon at the NIH in order to further study the great potential of stem cells.

PRESENT USE OF iPSCs FOR MEDICINE

How can iPSCs and ESCs improve medicine at this point in time? Generating patient-specific stem cells already has therapeutic potential. When a stem cell is derived from a patient with a disease, these stem cells allow us to investigate the mechanisms of that disease. Disease modeling also allows us to screen different drugs for a possible cure. In this way, different drugs are not tested on the whole patient, but only on the abnormal cells from the patient. Once a promising drug is selected, then clinical trials can begin in order to determine whether the drug can cure the patient (Figure 7.4, Table 7.1).

An example of this process is found in the work of Lee and colleagues in 2009 on a rare genetic disorder of the peripheral nervous system called familial dysautonomia (Lee et al. 2009). The disease is caused by a single point mutation in the gene encoding the inhibitor of the nuclear factor–κβ(IκB)–kinase complex-associated protein (IκBKAP). With the successful derivation of iPSCs from the patients with familial dysautonomia, the investigators were able to duplicate some of the disease pathogenesis in the iPSCs and then screen compounds in order to normalize cell behavior. They found that kinetin, a plant hormone, could partially normalize these diseased cells.

In cardiology, other investigators created iPSCs that were cardiac myocytes from individuals who have long-QT syndrome, which is an inheritable disease

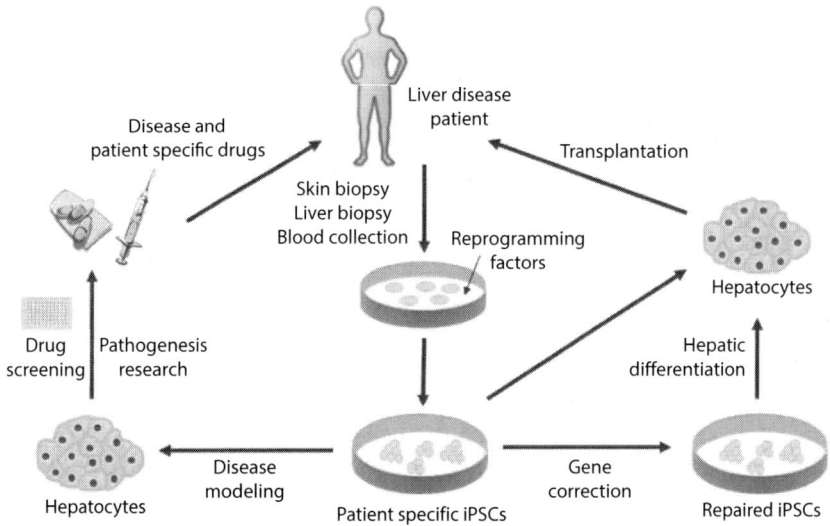

Figure 7.4 A possible application of human induced pluripotent stem cells for liver disease. Induced pluripotent stem cell technology from a specific patient can be used in gene therapy, cell replacement therapy, and modeling of a disease from that patient in order to discover possible drugs that could treat the patient. (Adapted from Chun, YS, P Chaudhari, and Y-Y Jang. 2010. *Int J Biol Sci* 6(7):796–805.)

associated with prolonged QT interval on an electrocardiogram and causes tachyarrhythmia of the heart that can lead to death. The QT interval is the time between the start of the Q wave and the end of the T wave in the heart's electrical cycle, involving electrical depolarization and repolarization of the ventricles of the heart. The disease is due to mutations in the KCNQ1 gene, which encodes the repolarizing potassium channel, mediating the electrical current in the heart. These investigators identified the cell defect and determined which drugs exacerbated the condition and which drugs improved function (Moretti et al. 2010).

The prolonged QT studies demonstrated that iPSC models could be used in order to identify cardiotoxic and beneficial effects of drugs in heart disease. Some of the questions that remain are: how many patients and how many iPSC lines must be created from patients in order to truly understand the disease process and determine a cure for any group of patients with a similar disease? However, it is apparent that ESC and iPSC technologies will be very helpful in disease modeling, drug discovery, and eventually autologous cell replacement therapies.

STEM CELLS AND PARKINSON'S DISEASE AND MACULAR DEGENERATION

Cell replacement therapies have been used in Parkinson's disease models with promising results. Parkinson's disease is characterized by progressive degeneration and death of dopaminergic (DA) neurons in the substantia nigra pars compacta of the brain, resulting in muscle rigidity, tremors, bradykinesia (slowness in the execution of movement), and akinesia (decreased bodily movement). Although there are drugs to alleviate some of these symptoms, the present pharmacotherapy cannot halt the progression of the disease and the loss of the DA neurons, nor can patients recover those neurons that have died. Stem cell transplantation therapy has shown some promise for patients with Parkinson's disease.

The first clinical trial for Parkinson's disease occurred in 1987 using aborted human fetal ventral midbrain tissue (Brundin et al. 1987). More than 400 patients with Parkinson's disease have been treated as part of this clinical trial so far. Some patients have exhibited dramatic improvements in their symptoms (Nishimura and Takahashi 2013). However, due to the religious issues surrounding the use of fetal tissue, this work has been hindered from progressing rapidly. So, scientists have used ESC and/or iPSC methodologies in order to generate midbrain DA neurons from pluripotent stem cells. In 2005, Takagi et al. demonstrated that primate ESC-derived DA neurons survive in a neurotoxin-treated primate model (the neurotoxin being 1-methyl-4-phenyl-1,2,2,6-tetrahydropyridine [MPTP]) for Parkinson's disease. These treated monkeys also had improved neurological scores and functional abilities compared to the sham-operated monkeys (Takagi et al. 2005). Human ESC-derived DA neurons have been generated and used in different animal models of Parkinson's disease, but several issues, such as the possibility of tumorigenicity, are obstacles to clinical trials (Nishimura and Takahashi 2013). However, there is still hope that these pitfalls will be overcome in the future to help Parkinson's disease patients.

Another promising result of hESC research is found in recent studies with hESC RPE that had been engineered in order to improve vision in patients with age-related macular degeneration and Stargardt's macular dystrophy. Both diseases cause blindness due to degeneration of the RPE, which leads to photoreceptor loss. Eighteen patients had hESCs derived from line MA09 cells—which had *ex vivo* exposure with mouse embryo cells and is thus classified as a xenotransplantation product—transplanted into one of their eyes after surgery (Schwartz et al. 2012). After 22 months of follow-up, no adverse proliferation, tissue rejection, or serious ocular or systemic safety issues were found, but some patients experienced minor issues (Schwartz et al. 2015). All patients had improved vision compared to their untreated eye. This study was the first evidence of medium-term safety, graft survival from hESC transplantation, and improved visual function for patients with eye diseases.

An incredible story of stem cells' ability to regenerate neural tissue has created hope for people disabled by spinal cord injuries (Paddock 2014). Mr. Darek Fidyka, a 40-year-old man, was left paralyzed from the chest down after a stab wound to his back in 2010. Dr. Geoffrey Raisman, a Professor of Neurology at University Hospital in the United Kingdom, had discovered that damaged nerve cells can form new connections to other nerve cells and had identified a type of nose cell, an olfactory ensheathing cell (OEC), which would allow neurons to regenerate into the brain. The OEC was used since it is the only known nerve cell capable of regenerating. The work of Dr. Raisman fascinated Dr. Pawel Tabakow, an Assistant Professor in Neurosurgery at Wroclaw University in Poland. He corresponded with Dr. Raisman and invited him to Poland, where they were able to transplant nasal OECs from each of three paraplegic patients into their own spinal cords. Mr. Fidyka was a recipient of this novel procedure using OECs and ankle nerve grafts in order to allow the OECs to bridge the gap caused by the spinal cord injury. After several surgeries and five hours a day of intensive rehabilitation with Dr. Tabakow, Darek Fidyka has sensation in his legs and is able to walk again, with the hope of soon being able to drive and live more independently. One of the reasons for the success of the surgery was that Darek's injury was a clean cut to his spinal cord; however, his case brings hope to the more than three million people worldwide who have spinal cord injuries, and illustrates the powerful potential of stem cells for regenerative medicine.

On a lighter side, this story reminds me of an old Woody Allen movie, *Sleeper*, and the cloning of the nose to bring back the leader of the organization. Who knew that movie was not so far-fetched in fantasy?

It is hoped that ESC and iPSC technologies will be used to improve neural and vascular function in many different types of patients in the future. Neurodegenerative diseases such as Parkinson's disease, which worsen with age, may benefit from neuron regeneration through iPSC technologies. Patients with Alzheimer's disease, which is characterized by increased amyloid plaques and neurofibrillary tangles in the brain, may be candidates for iPSC technology in order to regenerate normal neural tissue. Hepatitis C virus-induced liver cirrhosis can progress to liver cancer. If iPSC technologies can be used to regenerate the liver, then this disease could also be eradicated. Chronic kidney disease and end-stage renal failure may also benefit from iPSC technologies. In the future, we would replace damaged tissues with iPSCs generated from normal tissues in the patient and create true personalized medicine.

REFERENCES

Amabile, G and A Meissner. 2009. Induced pluripotent stem cells: Current progress and potential for regenerative medicine. *Trends Mol Med* 15:59–68.

Briggs, R and TJ King. 1952. Transplantation of living nuclei from blastula cells into enucleated frogs' eggs. *Proc Natl Acad Sci USA* 38:455–63.

Brundin, P, RE Strecker, O Lindvall et al. 1987. Intracerebral grafting of dopamine neurons. Experimental basis for clinical trials in patients with Parkinson's disease. *Ann N Y Acad Sci* 495:473–96.

Chun, YS, P Chaudhari, and Y-Y Jang. 2010. Applications of patient-specific induced pluripotent stem cells; focused on disease modeling, drug screening and therapeutic potentials for liver disease. *Int J Biol Sci* 6(7):796–805.

Evans, MJ and MH Kaufman. 1981. Establishment in culture of pluripotent cells from mouse embryos. *Nature* 292:154–6.

Gropp, M, V Shilo, G Vainer et al. 2012. Standardization of the teratoma assay for analysis of pluripotency of human ES cells and biosafety of their differentiated progeny. *PLoS One* 7(9):e45532.

Gurdon, JB. 1962. Adult frogs derived from the nuclei of single somatic cells. *Dev Biol* 4:256–73.

Isobe, K-I, Z Cheng, N Nishio, T Suganya, Y Tantaka, and S Ito. 2014. iPSCs, aging and age-related diseases. *New Biotech* 35(1):411–21.

Kim, K, A Doi, B Wen et al. 2010. Epigenetic memory in induced pluripotent stem cells. *Nature* 16:467(7313):285–90.

Laurent, LC, I Ulitsky, I Slavin et al. 2011. Dynamic changes in the copy number of pluripotency and cell proliferation genes in human ESCs and iPSCs during reprogramming and time in culture. *Cell Stem Cell* 8(1):106–18.

Lee, G, EP Papapetrou, H Kim et al. 2009. Modelling pathogenesis and treatment of familial dysautonomia using patient-specific iPSCs. *Nature* 17:461(7262):402–6.

Martin, GR. 1981. Isolation of a pluripotent cell line from early mouse embryos cultured in medium conditioned by teratocarcinoma stem cells. *Proc Natl Acad Sci USA* 78(12):7634–8.

Mayshar, Y, U Ben-David, N Lavon, JC Biancotti, B Yakir, AT Clark, K Plath, WE Lowry, and N Benvenisty. 2010. Identification and classification of chromosomal aberrations in human induced pluripotent stem cells. *Cell Stem Cell* 7(4):521–31.

Moretti, A, M Bellin, A Welling et al. 2010. Patient-specific induced pluripotent stem-cell models for long-QT syndrome. *N Engl J Med* 363(15):1397–409.

Nishimura, K and J Takahashi. 2013. Therapeutic application of stem cell technology toward the treatment of Parkinson's disease. *Biol Pharm Bull* 36(2):171–5.

Paddock, C. October 21, 2014. Medical New Today. http://www.medicalnews today.com.

Papp, B and K Plath. 2013. Epigenetics of reprogramming to induced pluripotency. *Cell* 152:1324–43.

Park, IH, R Zhao, JA West, A Yabuuchi, H Huo, TA Ince, PH Lerou, MW Lensch, and GQ Daley. 2008. Reprogramming of human somatic cells to pluripotency with defined factors. *Nature* 451(7175):141–6.

Robinton, DA and GQ Daley. 2012. The promise of induced pluripotent stem cells in research and therapy. *Nat Med* 481:295–305.

Schwartz, SD, J-P Hubschman, G Heilwell, V Franco-Cardenas, CK Pan, RM Ostrick, E Mickunas, R Gay, I Klimanskaya, and R Lanza. 2012. Embryonic stem cell trials for macular degeneration: A preliminary report. *Lancet* 379:713–20.

Schwartz, SD, CD Regillo, BL Lam et al. 2015. Human embryonic stem cell-derived retinal pigment epithelium in patients with age-related macular degeneration and Stargardt's macular dystrophy: Follow-up of two open-label phase 1/2 studies. *Lancet* 385:509–16.

Takagi, Y, J Takahashi, H Saiki et al. 2005. Dopaminergic neurons generated from monkey embryonic stem cells function in a Parkinson primate model. *J Clin Invest* 115(1):102–9.

Takahashi, K, K Tanabe, M Ohnuki, M Narita, T Ichisaka, K Tomoda, and S Yamanaka. 2007. Induction of pluripotent stem cells from adult human fibroblasts by defined factors. *Cell* 131(5):861–72.

Takahashi, K and S Yamanaka. 2006. Induction of pluripotent stem cells from mouse embryonic and adult fibroblast cultures by defined factors. *Cell* 126(4):663–76.

Yu, J, MA Vodyanik, K Smuga-Otto et al. 2007. Induced pluripotent stem cell lines derived from human somatic cells. *Science* 318(5858):1917–20.

Zhao, T, ZN Zhang, S Rong, and Y Xu. 2011. Immunogenicity of induced pluripotent stem cells. *Nature* 474:212–5.

8

Scientific studies and medical trials

Which type of scientific study or trial can best determine whether a particular therapy/drug will cure?

Can the illness or death of one person change the course of medicine? Figure 8.1 is a haunting picture of just such a person. Libby Zion died at the age of 18 in 1984 and the cause of her death was never found. She was an 18-year-old college student who was admitted to the hospital with a high fever, dehydration, and mysterious jerking movements (Lerner 2009). She had a history of depression and was taking phenelzine, an antidepressant. At that time, the diagnosis was that she probably had a viral infection. The resident on duty with the verbal permission from her family physician and the attending doctor on record agreed to give her meperidine, an opiate, to stop her shaking. However, Libby became more agitated, so the first-year resident on call, who did not visually examine her because she was so busy with other patients and understaffed, with the second-year resident having gone across the street for a few hours of rest, ordered physical restraint as well as haloperidol, another sedating medication. Records show that Libby calmed down. When her vitals were rechecked in the morning, she had a temperature of 107°. The staff tried to cool her body, but she went into cardiac arrest and died. When her father found out that Libby had been tied down, neglected until morning, and the only doctors who had seen her were doctors in training (i.e., residents), he was furious. He sued the hospital and started a campaign to reform the medical system. Residents at that time routinely worked 36-hour shifts, often with little or no sleep. Libby's story spread around the country. In the trial of 1994, the verdict placed equal blame on the hospital and Libby Zion, who had concealed her past use of cocaine. Ultimately, her death resulted in a change in resident work hours, workloads, and supervision. In 1987, Dr. Bertrand Bell, head of a New York State Commission, recommended that doctors-in-training (i.e., residents) work no more than 80 hours a week and no more than 24 hours in a row, and receive more on-site supervision from senior physicians. In 2003, the Accreditation Council for Graduate Medical Education made these recommendations mandatory for all residency training programs.

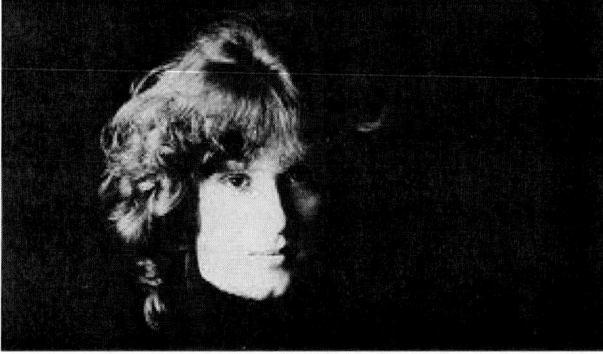

Figure 8.1 Picture of Libby Zion, who died at the age of 18 while in a hospital. Ultimately, her death resulted in a change in resident work hours, workloads, and supervision in hospitals. (Data from http://www.newmedicalterms.com/libby-zion/. Accessed on March 6, 2016.)

This story starts this chapter because personal stories and individual medical cases (case reports) can change the course of medical treatment. However, medicine relies mainly on the results from larger scientific trials such as randomized controlled trials (RCTs) that enroll many patients in order to determine whether a treatment or pharmaceutical is efficacious for a particular disease. A pitfall in personalized medicine is determining the best type and design of scientific/clinical trials. Much of personalized medicine may only pertain to a small group of patients. As such, how would we know what type of treatment is best for this small group when drug/treatment results rely on data from the responses of a large group of patients in order to determine statistical significance and any complications that would prevent this medication from being used routinely? If we personalize medicine, what will be the cost of these smaller trials and the cost of personalized medicine for our medical system in the United States, which is already the second most expensive medical system in the world? Finally, returning to the true story above, how should medical education and training be changed in order to address a shift in medical approach to personalized medicine?

CASE REPORTS

The true story of Libby Zion is not a case report, but it does show how one person and a concerned parent can change medicine. A case report is a detailed medical report of the symptoms, diagnosis, treatment, and follow-up of an individual patient who has an unusual disease or novel medical problem. Case reports can also contain a literature review of other related cases. A number of medical journals publish case reports, but not all clinical journals. In the history of medicine, there have been a number of seminal case reports. In fact, the value of case reports has been touted as being important as a first report of adverse drug reactions that are then confirmed by other physicians and lead to a more comprehensive study (Aronson and Hauben 2006).

Perhaps one of the most famous case reports was a letter published by the Australian obstetrician William McBride in *The Lancet* in 1961, in which he reported from his own practice of medicine that one in five women who had used a new drug to relieve morning sickness in early pregnancy had given birth to a severely deformed child: the babies had missing limbs (Vandenbroucke 2001). Two weeks earlier, the drug thalidomide had been removed from the market in the United Kingdom. It took years and many other reports, especially in the media, before the German company, Contergan, removed thalidomide from the drug market. Throughout the world, about 10,000 such cases were reported, especially in Europe, and only 50% of these children survived. Today, thalidomide is used only for some cancers and leprosy. Even today, the precise mechanism is not known regarding its immunomodulatory effects, which involve suppression of some cytokines along with antiangiogenic effects. We do know that thalidomide binds to and inactivates cereblon, an important protein in limb development, which was one of the reasons for the birth defects it caused.

Another type of case report that has greatly affected medicine is surgical cases. The following famous case report started with these words: "On December 3, 1967, a heart from a cadaver was successfully transplanted into a 54 year old man to replace a heart irreparably damaged by repeated myocardial infarction" (Benjamin and Barnes 2014). Dr. Christiaan Barnard in the Department of Surgery at the University of Cape Town and Groote Schumur Hospital, Cape Town, South Africa, was the author of this case report, which described the patient he had operated on, the operative technique, and postoperative care of the patient (Barnard 1967). Dr. Barnard's work was instrumental to doctors realizing that successful heart transplants were possible, and it provided them with the framework for further advances in cardiology.

Of course, not all case reports have led to important discoveries, but they are accepted as a means by which physicians can describe a successful, novel treatment of a patient, a possible drug complication, or a medical mystery. A case report, in general, gives poor evidence-based, statistically relevant medical proof, but if the finding is novel and interesting, then formal verification through more robust clinical trials, such as through a RCT, can then be justified and funded, with the enrollment of many more patients with a similar issue.

RCTs

The RCT is a type of scientific study in which patients are randomly allocated to different treatments under study, and it is considered the gold standard for a clinical trial (Figure 8.2). Subjects are recruited and assessed for eligibility for the study and then randomly assigned to treatment or control groups before the intervention begins, such as taking a specific new drug or undergoing novel surgery or another type of procedure. After randomization, the patients are followed

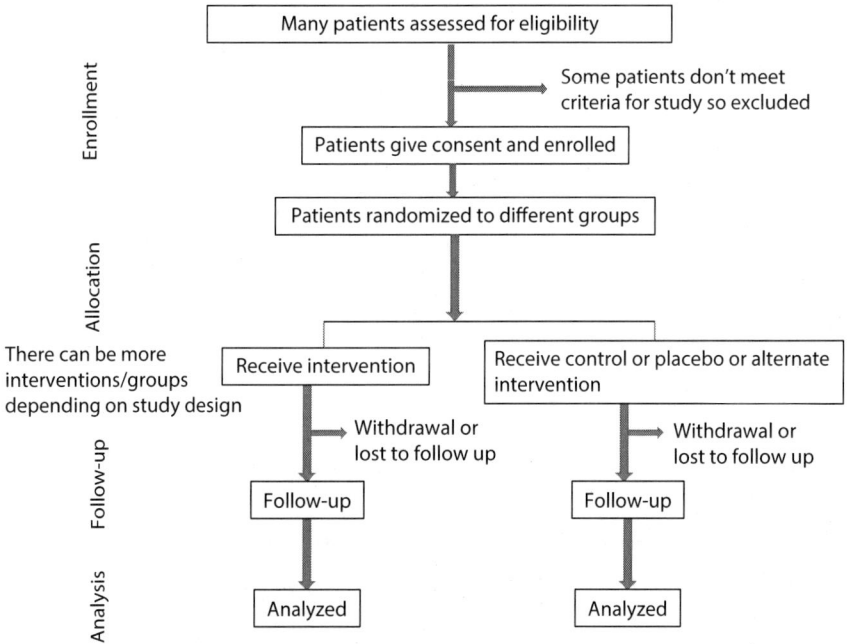

Figure 8.2 Flow chart of a sample randomized controlled trial. There are four phases of study design in a randomized controlled trial: enrollment of patients; random allocation of patients into intervention groups (for example, taking a specific drug or a placebo drug); follow-up of patients; and analysis of the data obtained from the study of these patients.

in exactly the same manner. The RCT term is used for studies that contain a control group, such as no treatment and/or placebo and/or a previously tested treatment (positive control). Not all randomized clinical trials are RCTs because, in some cases, controls would be impractical or unethical to institute. As of 2004, more than 150,000 RCTs were in the Cochrane library (a subscription-based database). To improve reporting of these RCTs in the medical literature, an international group of scientists and editors published Consolidated Standards of Reporting Trials (CONSORT) in 1996, 2001, and 2010 in order to keep track of these expensive but important types of trials that may lead to new treatment regimens in medicine.

An example of a successful RCT was a study in which doctors compared two classes of medications used for patients with arthritis and rheumatoid arthritis (Silverstein et al. 2000). Conventional nonsteroidal anti-inflammatory drugs (NSAIDs), such as aspirin, are known to have deleterious gastrointestinal (GI) effects; therefore, NSAIDs were compared to a drug, celecoxib, with the hypothesis that it would cause fewer GI effects such as ulcers. NSAIDs inhibit cyclooxygenase (COX), an enzyme that converts arachidonic acid (an endogenous type of fatty acid/lipid) into prostaglandins. COX exists in two forms: COX-1 and COX-2. Prostaglandins are a group of lipid compounds derived from fatty acids, are found in almost every tissue in humans and other animals, and have diverse functions such as vasodilation, contraction of smooth muscle, and a role in inflammation. COX-1 produces prostaglandins, which are responsible for the maintenance of GI mucosal integrity (the lining of the GI tract). COX-2 is a cyto-kine-induced enzyme that produces prostaglandins that mainly mediate pain and inflammation. NSAIDs inhibit both COX-1 and COX-2 to different degrees. Celecoxib only inhibits COX-2. Over 8000 patients in 386 clinical sites in the United States and Canada were enrolled for this RCT. Their results showed that fewer patients on celecoxib had GI blood loss, hepatotoxicity, GI intolerance, or renal toxicity than with NSAIDs.

The advantages of randomization in RCTs are the elimination of bias in treatment assignment. RCTs allow for a more objective analysis or blinding because the investigators and participants do not know the difference between the control and the treatment until the end of the study. However, in some cases, blinding is impossible if a new surgical approach, physical therapy, implant, etc., is being tested. Finally, RCTs allow the use of probability theory in order to determine whether the new medical approach is better than chance.

However, there are pitfalls with RCTs. If the sample size (i.e., patient group) is too small or not representative of the patient population, then definitive conclusions on the efficacy of a particular treatment cannot be made. Most RCTs are expensive to perform—costing many millions of dollars—and it often takes years for the results to be obtained and then published. Sometimes there are conflicts of interest with the investigators having ties to the pharmaceutical or medical company whose product is being tested, even though they are required to disclose these ties. Often the RCT may include patients whose prognosis is better with fewer serious health issues, which is not reflective of the true patient population; or the design of the RCT, reflecting the best care, would be difficult to implement on a large scale for all patients in different parts of the country or in other countries. Finally, there can be incomplete reporting of adverse effects, even though most institutions require these reports.

In 2000, two studies were published in the prestigious *New England Journal of Medicine* that found that observational studies and RCTs produced, in general, the same results (Benson and Hartz 2000; Concato et al. 2000). Observational studies are defined as either cohort studies (i.e., concurrent selection of controls) or a case–control design with clinical intervention and outcome. Another meta-analysis in 2001 studied 45 different topics and compared 240 RCTs and 168 nonrandomized studies, and found that seven RCTs had a small but significant increase in the magnitude of treatment effect compared to nonrandomized studies.

OTHER TYPES OF MEDICAL STUDIES AND THE ISSUES WITH RCTs

The consensus in medicine is that when study designs are ranked by their potential for new discoveries, anecdotal evidence would be first, followed by observational studies, and then RCTs. Of course, anecdotal evidence, such as in a case study, needs to be further explored with more patients, rigorous statistics, and appropriate controls, but they often lead to more exploration of a new topic. In some situations, RCTs may be unnecessary for a treatment that has a dramatic and rapid effect. This happened with combination chemotherapy for metastatic testicular cancer, which increased the cure rate from 5% to 60% in a nonrandomized study (Einhorn 2002; Wittes 2002). Thus, the benefit was so significant that additional studies were not needed. Often it is a doctor's (both PhDs and MDs) initial observations that spur them to study a topic in more detail through a more scientific approach in a funded study, and then in a RCT.

For personalized medicine, RCTs become difficult to perform, because the number of patients with identical individual needs becomes smaller for selection and analysis. Multiple smaller studies become more expensive to perform, and the benefit for a few patients may not be considered adequate to justify funding the study. The greatest issue is determining the mathematical significance of these findings in a small study. In addition, the findings may be applied to other patients without the strict criteria that were followed when the new protocol or drug was tested in that small group of subjects. This could lead to a higher risk to patients. Bioinformatics may find a better approach to deal with this new problem. For example, meta-analysis is a statistical technique for combining the findings from independent studies in order to determine the clinical effectiveness for the larger population.

RCTs may not be appropriate for testing everything of health benefit. For example, in Western science, we have taken the approach of isolating and testing one active ingredient. However, there are examples in which a combination of factors is necessary for improved medical outcome. Funding organizations do not like to fund research on multiple ingredients without knowledge of what each one does separately. The beneficial effect may be lost, since each factor in the compound may interact and/or counterbalance the other to promote health.

An example of studying several components within a naturally occurring herb versus the one essential ingredient in it is feverfew. Feverfew is a plant that has been traditionally used for fevers, migraine headaches, rheumatoid arthritis, stomach aches, and even insect bites. Much of its activity has been attributed to one of its active compounds: parthenolide. The National Center for Complementary and Integrative Medicine (NCCIM; previously named the National Center for Complementary and Alternative Medicine [NCCAM]) on their website says that there is not enough evidence to assess any of feverfew's beneficial effects and mentions negative results from research trials on its effects without citing in which studies these results were found. On the other hand, if you turn to the website of the Memorial Sloan Kettering Cancer Institute in New York City, they list the evidence for a parthenolide-free extract of feverfew demonstrating free radical-scavenging properties, which is helpful against UV-induced sun damage. Another study shows that feverfew has antiprotozoal properties, and a feverfew extract reduced the frequency of migraine headaches in a clinical trial. However, before you can access this information on the Memorial Sloan Kettering Cancer Institute website, you have to agree to the following statement: "Memorial Sloan Kettering Cancer Center makes no warranties nor express or implied representations whatsoever regarding the accuracy, completeness, timeliness, comparative or controversial nature, or usefulness of any information contained or referenced on this Web site. Memorial Sloan Kettering does not assume any risk whatsoever for your use of this website or the information contained herein" (http://www.mskcc.org, January 27, 2015).

Are these two sets of results ambiguous due to differences in the preparation of feverfew, with extracts of feverfew having only one or two of the active ingredients necessary for all of its beneficial results, or does extraction lead to inactivating of the essential factors for its activity? Many scientists are now suggesting that many herbals and botanicals have beneficial effects due to a number of compounds in the natural product that potentiate and balance its multiple effects. One job the NCCIM has taken on is to try and standardize extracts from herbals, such as feverfew, so that researchers can perform studies with them and be able to compare their results in order to determine effects in a consistent manner. However, it is important that research should not be directed at only finding the one "active ingredient" that may not be the ingredient by which the botanical or herbal medicine acts. We need to be more broad-minded and not study the benefits of an herbal/botanical only to find the one ingredient that can be developed further by pharmaceutical companies and then marketed.

Scientists often will not fund research on topics for which there is not a mechanism, and they demonstrate bias for what they require as a mechanism. For example, research funds were slow to fund studies in integrative medicine research such as acupuncture, not to mention studies on a topic such as energy medicine—that is, human biofield studies—a topic that has been totally ignored and banned from the NCCIM website. Acupuncture is now accepted as a treatment for certain types of pain (see Chapter 5). On the other hand, aspirin is accepted as a therapeutic treatment without knowing the mechanisms underlying all of its actions. Aspirin is a common over-the-counter drug that has a number of detrimental effects that have been recently found. Scientists have discovered that excessive use of aspirin causes GI bleeding, so it cannot be taken like candy and needs to be monitored by a doctor. Only after excessive use of aspirin was it found that children under the age of 16 years should not be prescribed aspirin for influenza-like symptoms or viral illnesses because of the risk of Reye's syndrome in some young patients. Reye's syndrome can be fatal and is detrimental to the brain and liver, and also causes low blood sugar, but the exact mechanisms underlying these effects are not known. In conclusion, routine use of aspirin needs to be monitored by a doctor.

We cannot demand that only those therapies deemed effective by an RCT be accepted for medical treatment. Even RCTs are fallible. For example, the implantable cardioverter–defibrillator (ICD) therapy studies were very controversial (Revenco et al. 2011). Presently, over 40% of new ICD implants for heart failure are given to patients who are over 70 years old. However, the original RCTs had no age requirements, since the main criterion for patient selection was heart failure with a heart ejection fraction of less than 35%. Sudden cardiac death occurs mostly in younger patients with heart failure, while older patients die from progressive heart failure and bradyarrhythmias (very slow and irregular heartbeats). We now know that the ICD is of benefit to younger patients, who have an increased risk of sudden cardiac death, but in the early RCTs, their findings were applied to all ages of patients. Finally, when age was analyzed in another RCT, entitled *"The Sudden Cardiac Death in Heart Failure Trial,"* patients older than 65 years did not demonstrate any benefit from ICDs compared to the placebo arm of the trial (Bardy et al. 2005). In another trial in which patients who were over 75 years old were analyzed (Healey et al. 2007), it was found that the older patient population had other comorbidities that needed to be considered, such as higher complications from surgery, higher mortality, and longer hospital stays that can be more debilitating for geriatric patients. "Thus, to date, no clear evidence exists for any beneficial role of the ICD in patients older than 75 years" (Revenco et al. 2011).

ANIMAL STUDIES

Another approach to studying drug responses and disease mechanisms is the use of cell and animal subjects. Many experiments cannot be performed on humans, since we are not sure of their outcome, which may be harmful or even cause death, unless we perform initial tests. Medicine cannot advance unless we acknowledge the sacrifices that many animals have made for knowledge leading to our own health and well-being. Mouse models have been the cornerstone of animal research, since genetic manipulation of mice through the addition of specific genes, even human genes (transgenic mice), or the removal of specific genes (knockouts) can be used in order to study the action of a specific gene or genes in the development or maintenance of any tissue (Figure 8.3). Most animal studies are performed on animals that are especially bred for research. Although there is a plethora of animal and cell studies, their findings need to be confirmed in humans. Human medical studies will always be the definitive test for determining the efficacy of a new medical procedure or drug and determining the mechanisms underlying a particular disease.

Due to the outcry against the maltreatment of animals in research, which has been spearheaded by non-scientists (that is, lay people) fighting for animal rights, academic institutions have strict guidelines for animal work. Lengthy applications for animal research protocols must be first approved by an impartial group of doctors and a lay person(s) on the institutional board for animal research. Animals are housed in separate facilities run by dedicated and trained staff with required procedures for housing and feeding along with environmental

Advantages and disadvantages of mouse models for scientific study

Advantages	Disadvantages
Genetic models can be created to study function of specific genes: transgenic, gene knock-out (KO), or knock-in	Transgene integration is random and can cause changes to other genes or to the gene of interest
Relatively inexpensive to breed, house, and work with mice, although transgenic rescue of a KO can be time-consuming, expensive, and labor intensive	Many genes are redundant or subtle in their differences in function so KO or transgenic mouse may not express obvious phenotypic changes
Mice are small, have large litters in a short time frame, and have an accelerated lifespan compared to humans. One mouse year is approximately 30 human years	Not enough comparative animal physiological studies on mouse versus human responses have been performed to validate all types of studies in mice
Mice are good models for human diseases or probing endocrine, nervous, cardiovascular, skeletal, and other mammalian physiological systems	Mice are poor models for (1) human inflammatory diseases, (2) trauma-related responses especially those also involving inflammatory system, and (3) burns
Mice heal fast and less susceptible to infection from surgical procedures than larger animals and humans	Mice are small so that some surgical procedures are difficult to perform
Drug testing in animals is often first performed on mice for the reasons above	For drugs to be approved larger animal models must be used and then testing with FDA approval in humans
Mice naturally develop diseases similar to human diseases such as cancer, atherosclerosis, hypertension, diabetes, osteoporosis, and glaucoma	Certain diseases do not afflict mice such as cystic fibrosis and Alzheimer's. However, some of these diseases can be induced by manipulating the mouse genome or environment

Figure 8.3 Advantages and disadvantages of mouse models for scientific study. Mouse models are the most extensive tool for the study of disease and cellular function, due to the ability to study specific genes and their functions through knocking out genes, knocking in genes, or creating transgenic mice. The advantages and disadvantages of mouse models are listed.

enrichment. Veterinarians are a part of most academic institution's facilities, along with other dedicated animal care specialists. Laboratories engaging in animal research are routinely evaluated for their procedures and physically inspected, and cannot deviate from their approved animal research application, or else their work with animals will be stopped, and their funding can even be rescinded. Many grant funding entities require specific institutional animal protocols and facilities before they will release funding for a study. These animal studies are very important for the advancement of science that can lead us to personalized medicine. However, the strict guidelines imposed on animal studies are necessary in order to prevent animal suffering and abuse.

Again, there are pitfalls in relying on just one type of study to answer a specific medical or scientific question. Recently, mouse models have been shown to be poor models (Figure 8.3) for mimicking human inflammatory diseases (particularly endotoxemia), trauma-related responses (especially involving the inflammatory system), and burns (Seok et al. 2013). Endotoxemia is caused by endotoxins, which are toxic substances that are part of a bacterium's cell wall and are released when the bacterium ruptures. Endotoxins are found in bacterial infections and can lead to severe medical symptoms and even death.

In contrast, a recent study was published showing the relationship between mice and humans in relation to the microbiota common in both species (Ridaura et al. 2013). The microbiota is the community of microorganisms that are found in our body (Figure 8.4). The human body contains more than 10 times more microbial cells than human cells. Recently (in the 1990s), the microbiota was

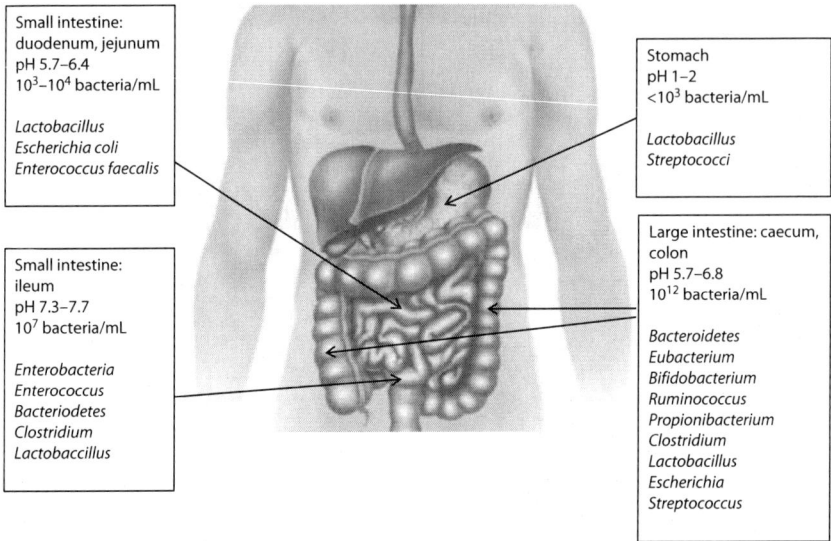

Small intestine:
duodenum, jejunum
pH 5.7–6.4
10^3–10^4 bacteria/mL

Lactobacillus
Escherichia coli
Enterococcus faecalis

Stomach
pH 1–2
$<10^3$ bacteria/mL

Lactobacillus
Streptococci

Small intestine:
ileum
pH 7.3–7.7
10^7 bacteria/mL

Enterobacteria
Enterococcus
Bacteriodetes
Clostridium
Lactobaccillus

Large intestine: caecum,
colon
pH 5.7–6.8
10^{12} bacteria/mL

Bacteroidetes
Eubacterium
Bifidobacterium
Ruminococcus
Propionibacterium
Clostridium
Lactobacillus
Escherichia
Streptococcus

Figure 8.4 Microbiota. The microbiota is the community of microorganisms that are found in or on our bodies. The human body contains more than 10 times more microbial cells than human cells, and these microbial cells play important roles in human health and disease, which has only recently been discovered. The figure of a person demonstrates where microbiota can be found in the gastrointestinal tract.

recognized as playing an important role in human health and disease. Microbiota can be found in the gut (GI tract), including the mouth, skin, and urogenital canals. In the study by Ridaura et al. (2013), human twins were studied in which one twin was obese and the other lean. Scientists transferred fecal gut bacteria—microbiota—from these humans into germ-free mice and demonstrated that mice with microbiota from the obese twins grew fat, while those from the lean twins stayed lean. The fat mice received food high in fat and low in fruits and vegetables, which kept the gut bacteria from the fat twins viable, and the mice remained fat. The thin twins' bacteria were maintained only if the mice received food pellets that were rich in fruits and vegetable and low in fat. Co-housing mice with the obese twins' microbiota with mice containing lean co-twin microbiota prevented the development of increased body mass. At this point, we do not understand the mechanism behind these results, except that it is related to specific members of the bacteria class Bacteroidetes from the lean twin's microbiota, but excitement is growing for developing diets that might change the gut bacteria of obese patients so that they can lose weight. Thus, studies with mice, humans, and bacteria can be designed in which important scientific information can be gleaned.

Most drug testing requires testing in animal models that are often mouse models initially and then larger animal models, before they are tested in humans. However, comparative physiological studies for specific animal versus human responses are necessary in order to validate results from animal studies. There are few published comparative animal studies.

CELL STUDIES

Isolated cells are another system that is important in biochemistry for studying signaling pathways that rule a cell's behavior and expression. The field of cell biology uses cell models in order to understand cellular functions. Biotechnology uses cells in order to test drugs and biomaterials for human use (Figure 8.5). Most often, immortalized cell lines from humans and animals are used. These cells have been mutated either naturally or intentionally in the laboratory, so that they can keep growing without going through the process of senescence and/ or death. Cellular senescence is a phenomenon by which normal diploid cells (a typical human diploid cell is a somatic cell that contains 46 chromosomes) cease to divide, which occurs in aging. A pitfall in using cell lines is that they are immortalized; therefore, they are not normal (i.e., cell death is normal). When we use cell lines, we cannot be sure that the cell process or gene we are studying is unaffected by immortalization.

Advantages and disadvantages of cell studies

Advantages	Disadvantages
Human cells from practically every tissue in the body can be grown and studied in the laboratory to understand human cell function and pathology	Cell interactions with other types of cells and with the extracellular environment in tissues cannot be reproduced to give an accurate picture of how these interactions affect cell function
Immortalized cell lines exist for most cell types and even primary cells can be immortalized, so that large volumes of cells can be propagated for many different studies Large amount of DNA, RNA, and proteins from cells can be isolated for analysis	Immortalized cell lines lose some of the functions of normal cells Spontaneous or induced random mutagenesis can occur in cell culture Primary human cells have a limited lifespan and lose their phenotype with passage in culture
Immortalized cell lines are widely used as a simple model for more complex biological systems, especially to study one or a few aspects of that complex system	Cells can be too simple for understanding the important aspects of the biological system of interest
Diseased cells can be compared to normal cells to understand the pathological change	Diseased cells may be heterogeneous in a tissue. Cell propagation in a laboratory may not reflect the true complexity of the disease and what factors are causing the pathological response. Endocrine and paracrine factors are absent in cell culture
Drug testing in cells can assess dosing and possible drug toxicity	A drug given systemically may be toxic to other cell types in a different tissue in the body
Cell signaling leading to the biological outcome of interest can be studied and targeted therapeutically	The laboratory culture environment may affect cell signaling pathways

Figure 8.5 Advantages and disadvantages of cell culture studies for scientific study. Human cells from practically every tissue can be grown and studied in the laboratory. The advantages and disadvantages of using human cells in order to study normal and pathologic processes are discussed.

An example of a cell line is HeLa, which is the oldest and most commonly used human cell line, derived from a 31-year-old African–American patient, Henrietta Lacks, who had cervical cancer. She died 8 months after a researcher, George Gey, isolated her cells. These cells were mass produced and have been used for research on AIDS, drug toxicity, cancer, gene mapping, radiation damage, etc. These cells were instrumental in the development of the polio vaccine in 1954 (Skloot 2010). Neither Lacks nor her family gave permission for researchers to harvest her cells, but at that time in the 1950s, procedures and policies on cell use from patients had not been developed. Rebecca Skloot, in her 2010 book, *The Immortal Life of Henrietta Lacks* (Skloot 2010), documented the history of the Lacks family and HeLa cells. The existence of these cells was hidden from members of the Lacks family and the family never received monetary benefit, unlike the doctors. A similar case, Moore versus Regents of the University of California, came before the Supreme Court of California in 1990. The court ruled that a person's discarded tissue is not the property of that individual. However, the research physician did have an obligation to reveal his/her financial interests in the harvested tissue, and the patient has the right to bring a claim and proof of injury as a result of the physician's failure to disclose. Today, written permission must be received from the patient to harvest any tissue for use in research purposes.

An underutilized approach in the scientific research in personalized medicine is to use normal human cells or primary cells that have been discarded after surgical procedures (Figure 8.6). Due to this being discarded tissue that would otherwise be thrown away, these tissues do not require permission from the patient for their propagation and use in scientific research. However, the researcher is not allowed to know who the tissue came from. The only information available is the cell source, general medical condition of the patient, sex, and age. Patient identification and names are kept confidential.

A pitfall for primary cell use is that such cells have a limited lifespan, similarly to all cells in our bodies. Another concern has been that primary cells are isolated from multicellular and multifunctional tissues, and may have other types of cells besides the cell type of interest, which could interfere with the interpretation of the results. However, we now have particular media for keeping cells alive in a culture dish under sterile conditions that promote the growth of only the cells of interest and inhibit the growth of other contaminating cells (Freshney 2010). Still, it is important to check the purity of the cell population being studied. With long periods of growth in the laboratory, these primary cells also lose the phenotypic expression of the cell type/tissue from which they were taken. Therefore, only a specific number of generations or cell passages can be used. On the other hand, these cells are personalized, since they are from a single individual.

Cell and tissues from human body

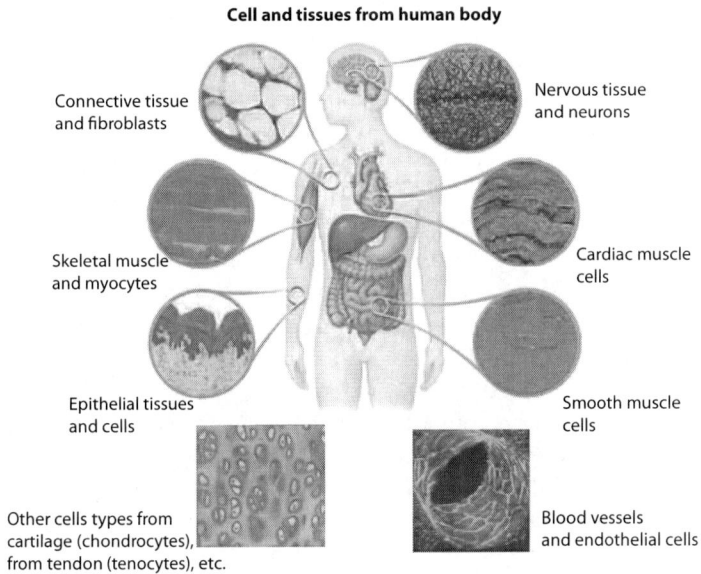

Connective tissue
and fibroblasts

Nervous tissue
and neurons

Skeletal muscle
and myocytes

Cardiac muscle
cells

Epithelial tissues
and cells

Smooth muscle
cells

Other cells types from
cartilage (chondrocytes),
from tendon (tenocytes), etc.

Blood vessels
and endothelial cells

Figure 8.6 A representation of some of the cell types that can be isolated from the human body and used for scientific study in the laboratory.

The study of particular cells from individuals with the same disease can be helpful in determining disease mechanisms, specific features of the cell that are affected by that disease, and even disease treatment, if the results are consistent across the patient population. The diseased cell can be compared to similar cells from healthy individuals in order to determine what is wrong and to assess whether a drug can correct the problem so that the diseased cell behaves normally. Thus, the use of primary cell cultures is a method that capitalizes on a personal approach, which may lead to important discoveries for personalized medicine.

My own research in tissue engineering and the compatibility of biomaterials has relied heavily on primary human cells. In one study, we used the bone cells (osteoblasts) from 102 patients of different ages undergoing elective orthopedic procedures in order to study the effects of age on the bone-forming capacity of these cells. We found that osteoblasts from female middle-aged and female older patients (above 60 years of age) had a reduced capacity to form bone compared to cells from younger patients and from all male patients (Zhang et al. 2004). These studies demonstrated age-dependent decreases in bone formation in older female patients. Older female patients may require additional therapeutic treatments in order to augment bone formation during fracture repair or implant placement. We also used primary osteoblast cultures in order to study the biocompatibility to various implant materials and so determine whether human bone cells will grow and form bone on novel implant materials (Ahmad et al. 1999; Sagomonyants et al. 2008, 2011).

In other bone studies, we have investigated the disease process in otosclerosis (Gronowicz et al. 2014). Otosclerosis is a focal disease of the human temporal bone, particularly the stapes bone. It is among the most common causes of acquired hearing loss in the United States, as it affects 0.1%–1% of the general population. We were able to compare osteoblasts from the stapes bone from patients with otosclerosis to the same type osteoblast from normal hearing patients and identify particular genes that may cause the hypermineralization of the stapes bone that leads to deafness (Gronowicz et al. 2014). In my laboratory we study bone, but many other scientists are using other types of human cells, such as neurons, lymphocytes, skin (epithelial), and tendon (tenocytes) cells, etc., in order to try and understand the cellular and genetic processes in the diseases affecting various tissues and even normal processes such as aging.

The hope for these animal and cell studies is to advance scientific understanding of disease processes and the genes and proteins that are not behaving normally. We cannot add or remove specific genes in humans with success at this point. Perhaps this will be a future scientific advancement, especially with the development of embryonic stem cell and induced pluripotent stem cell technology.

COMPUTER-BASED MODELING

Another important area of investigation is three-dimensional computer-based modeling, which has numerous applications in science. For example, this technique is used to anatomically map particular organs and tissues, either for understanding structural variability between patients or mapping surgical procedures. MRI-planned resections for tumors and amputations—in this case with osteosarcomas—changed after chemotherapy, so that surgeons needed to take this into consideration when basing their surgeries on pre-chemotherapy MRI images. Appropriate surgical procedures could then be planned (Jones et al. 2012). Other applications are computer-aided drug design and molecular modeling based on the x-ray crystal structure coordinates of proteins. In the future, computer modeling of complex genetic systems and for genomics will be helpful for understanding the vast array of data from genomic studies (Chen et al. 2014).

PEER REVIEW OF MEDICAL AND SCIENTIFIC STUDIES LEADING TO PUBLICATION

Extremely important to mention regarding any published scientific or medical article is the peer-review process that is required prior to publication. Once a scientific study is completed, it must be submitted to a journal of the authors' choice and will not be published until more than three doctors have read and reviewed its results, checking the methods to make sure that they are accurate, checking the statistics, and reviewing the results and the discussion of the results. If there is a group of authors who participated in the study, they must all sign a paper stating that they have reviewed the manuscript and agree with its findings. The authors must also disclose any ties with any agency or company that might prejudice their findings, and must reveal who funded their work. The reviewers have to agree that the paper is accurate and worthy of publication. Most studies are sent back with suggestions on how to improve the study. The work will not be published until the authors have adequately addressed the questions in a separate document, and made the necessary changes to their paper or have performed additional tests in order to make sure that their findings are accurate. Journals are ranked and the most prestigious journals usually have higher criteria for publication in their journal. It is very competitive and the process is believed to ensure the accuracy of the published studies so that a reader can determine that the results are evidence based and correct. Of course, if the results are confirmed in independent laboratories and published, then this increases the likelihood that the data and conclusions are correct. It is hoped that this rigorous process will provide readers with accurate data upon which to base their own studies and their own medical practice.

In conclusion, we need to rely on different types of scientific studies from cells, animals, and humans in order to understand the best treatments for patients. Only the test of time and multiple confirmatory results from different investigations in the scientific literature can point to the correct diagnosis and therapeutics. Personalizing medicine makes it more difficult, since conclusions on best medical practice can be difficult to assess from studies on individuals or small groups of patients with the tools we have available at this time. In addition, if the results from small studies are applied to other patients, this may increase health risks for these patients. Perhaps the best message is that we need to be open to all approaches in the medical literature and fund further research. There is value to all types of studies for elucidating the mechanisms underlying biological and physiological processes, for determining best treatment practices, and for improving health based on new evidence-based findings. Prejudice towards specific types of studies is wrong and the results from all types of studies must be evaluated for their efficacy by physicians and researchers. Evidence-based results should be evenly considered by physicians and scientists without personal bias and included in the medical curriculum.

REFERENCES

Ahmad, M, M-B McCarthy, and G Gronowicz. 1999. An *in vitro* model for mineralization of human osteoblast-like cells on implant materials. *Biomaterials* 20:211–20.

Aronson, JK and M Hauben. 2006. Drug safety: Anecdotes that provide definitive evidence. *BMJ* 333:1267–9.

Bardy, GH, KL Lee, DB Mark et al. 2005. Amiodarone or an implantable cardioverter–defibrillator for congestive heart failure. *N Engl J Med* 352(3):225–37.

Barnard, CN. 1967. A human cardiac transplant: An interim report of a human successful operation performed at Groote Schuur Hospital, Cape Town. *South African Med J* 41:1271–4.

Benjamin, SM and NC Barnes. 2004. Cardiac transplantation: Since the first case report specialty: Landmark case report; cardiothoracic surgery; transplantation article type: Original case report. *Grand Rounds* 4:L1–3.

Benson, K and AJ Hartz. 2000. A comparison of observational studies and randomized, controlled trials. *N Engl J Med* 342(25):1878–86.

Chen, HS, CM Hutter, LE Mechanic et al. 2014. Genetic simulation tools for post-genome wide association studies of complex diseases. *Genet Epidemiol* 39(1):11–9.

Concato, J, N Shah, and RI Horwitz. 2000. Randomized, controlled trials, observational studies, and the hierarchy of research designs. *N Engl J Med* 342(25):1887–92.

Einhorn, LH. 2002. Curing metastatic testicular cancer. *Proc Natl Acad Sci USA* 99(7):4592–5.

Freshney, IR. 2010. *Culture of Animal Cells: A Manual of Basic Technique and Specialized Applications*, 6th edition. Wiley-Blackwell, Hoboken, NJ.

Gronowicz, G, YL Richardson, J Flynn, J Kveton, M Eisen, G Leonard, M Aronow, C Rodner, and K Parham. 2014. Differences in otosclerotic and normal human stapedial osteoblast properties are normalized by alendronate *in vitro. Otolaryngol Head Neck Surg* 151(4):657–66.

Healey, JS, AP Hallstrom, KH Kuck, G Nair, EP Schron, RS Roberts, CA Morillo, and SJ Connolly. 2007. Role of the implantable defibrillator among elderly patients with a history of life-threatening ventricular arrhythmias. *Eur Heart J* 28(14):1746–9.

Jones, KB, PC Ferguson, B Lam, DJ Biau, S Hopyan, B Deheshi, AM Griffin, LM White, and JS Wunder. 2012. Surgeons can reliably record the anatomic details of a planned resection of an osteosarcoma. *J Bone Joint Surg Am* 94(15):1399–405.

Lerner, BH. 2009. A life-changing case for doctors in training. *New York Times*, March 3, 2009.

Revenco, D, JP Morgan, and L Tsao. 2011. The dilemma of implantable cardioverter–defibrillator therapy in the geriatric population. *J Geriatric Cardiol* 8:195–200.

Ridaura, VK, JJ Faith, FE Rey et al. 2013. Gut microbiota from twins discordant for obesity modulate metabolism in mice. *Science* 341(6150):1241214.

Sagomonyants, KB, M Hakim-Zargar, A Jhaveri, MS Aronow, and G Gronowicz. 2011. Porous tantalum stimulates the proliferation and osteogenesis of osteoblasts from elderly female patients. *J Orthop Res* 29(4):609–16.

Sagomonyants, KB, ML Jarman-Smith, JN Devine, MS Aronow, and GA Gronowicz. 2008. The *in vitro* response of human osteoblasts to polyetheretherketone (PEEK) substrates compared to commercially pure titanium. *Biomaterials* 29(11):1563–72.

Seok, J, HS Warren, AG Cuenca et al. 2013. Genomic responses in mouse models poorly mimic human inflammatory diseases. *Proc Natl Acad Sci USA* 110(9):3507–12.

Silverstein, FE, G Faich, JL Goldstein et al. 2000. Gastrointestinal toxicity with celecoxib vs nonsteroidal anti-inflammatory drugs for osteoarthritis and rheumatoid arthritis: The CLASS study: A randomized controlled trial. Celecoxib Long-term Arthritis Safety Study. *JAMA* 284(10):1247–55.

Skloot, R. 2010. *The Immortal Life of Henrietta Lacks*. New York: Random House.

Vandenbroucke, JP. 2001. In defense of case reports and case series. *Ann Intern Med* 134(4):330–4.

Wittes, J. 2002. Sample size calculations for randomized controlled trials. *Epidemiol Rev* 24(1):39–53.

Zhang, H, CG Lewis, MS Aronow, and G Gronowicz. 2004. The effects of patient age on human osteoblasts' response to Ti-6A1-4V implants *in vitro*. *J Orthop Res* 22:30–38.

9

Medical training for personalized medicine

How do we best teach our medical students, residents, and physicians to evaluate clinical data from studies such as randomized controlled trials (RCTs)? With the plethora of medical–scientific studies and evidence, how do we teach them the best course of treatment for their patients in a personalized medicine system?

Medical education is lagging behind the rapid advances in the sciences of genomics, epigenetics, proteomics, integrative medicine, etc., upon which personalized medicine will be based. In general, the medical school curriculum is 4 years in duration, with 2 years of basic training in science and medicine and then 2 years of clinical experiences (Figure 9.1) in Liaison Committee on Medical Education (LCME)–accredited U.S. medical schools, consisting of preclinical and clinical parts. After completing medical school, students earn their doctor of medicine degrees (MDs), although often they must complete additional training before practicing on their own as physicians.

Medical school education is filled with material that is the foundation of medical practice with little time to spare for other topics. When they leave medical school as MDs, doctors need to have a firm understanding of the basics in medicine for application to the population at large before they can start learning how to tailor treatments for individual patients. Through a national matching program, newly graduated MDs enter into a residency program that is 3–7 years or more of professional training under the supervision of senior physician educators. The length of residency training varies depending on the medical specialty chosen; for example, family practice, internal medicine, and pediatrics require 3 years of training, while general surgery requires 5 years.

For personalized medicine, doctors need to know which tests to perform in order to obtain more personalized information on a patient's condition. Then, knowledge of different treatment modalities is needed that is specific to a patient's condition. Then, some patients may require tailored therapies because

Typical medical school timeline

| Undergraduate education (4 years) | Medical school (4 years) | Residency (2 years) | Fellowship (1–2 years) |

| Take medical school prerequisites | Years 1 and 2: General medical education (usually in the classroom) | Year 3: Clinical education (Rotations) | Year 4: Specialty electives and residency apps | (Optional) Further study of a specialty |

| MCAT Admissions test | USMLE Step 1: Test over first 2 years of study | USMLE Step 2: Clinical test | USMLE Step 3: Clinical test | Board exams |

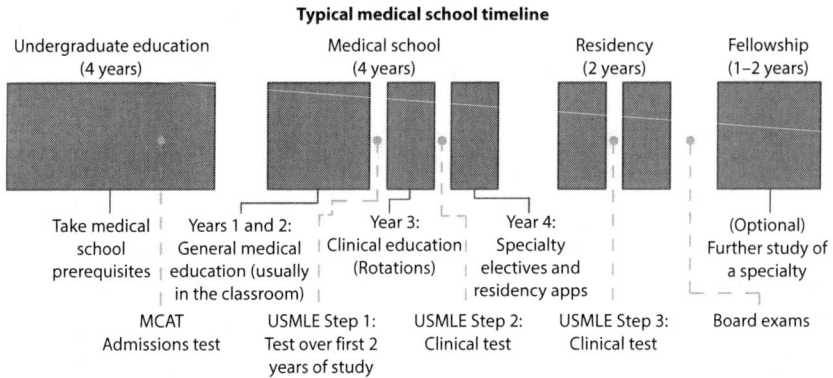

Figure 9.1 Timetable for medical education. In college, an undergraduate must take the prerequisite courses for medical school admission and the Medical College Admission Test® (MCAT®). Medical school is usually 2 years of general, basic medical education in the classroom and then 2 more years of clinical work. At the end of their second year, medical students take the U.S. Medical Licensing Examination® (USMLE®) step 1 examination. The second step of the USLME examination occurs after the third year of medical school. The final USMLE test occurs after the first year of residency, and further determines a doctor's knowledge of clinical practice. Some residencies, such as orthopedics, are 4 years in duration. Board examinations in the physician's chosen specialty are taken after their residency in order to determine their proficiency in their specialty. Further study in a specialty is optional.

of their genetics and/or physiological traits. With a more tailored and complicated scenario for personalizing medical diagnosis and treatment, the majority of personalized medicine may best be taught with more depth in residency training (LaChance and Murphy 2014).

GENOMICS AND THE MEDICAL SCHOOL CURRICULUM

At this point, there is no consensus on how physicians should be trained in practicing personalized medicine, and little literature exists on the best approach for curriculum changes. However, much of personalized medicine will be based upon an individual's genes. Therefore, basic genetic principles and epigenetics, exposure to a range of patients with genetic diseases, and learning to interpret clinical diagnostic assays based on biochemical, molecular, and genetic techniques can be the start of the intellectual foundation for personalized medicine (Dhar et al. 2012).

Less than 10 years ago, genomics was not routinely covered in medical schools, so we have a great deal of catch-up to do in educating physicians. For example, in a recent study, 153 medical and osteopathic schools in the United States and Canada were sent a questionnaire on genetics curricula (Plunkett-Rondeau et al. 2015). Most schools taught genetics in the first 2 years of medical school, but only

26% reported formal genetics teaching in the last 2 years of school. Most teachers felt that the amount of time spent on genetics was inadequate for preparing physicians for clinical practice. Medical students also need to be made aware of community and patient advocacy groups in order to help their patients with particular genetic conditions, and they must be allowed to author or present scholarly work on genomics and personalized medicine so that they are familiar with the topics that are the bases of personalized medicine. Interestingly, Japan is developing genomics curricula that start as early as high school in order to prepare for personalized medicine (Narimatsu et al. 2013).

A number of other topics have also been added to medical school curricula: personalized medicine (21%), direct-to-consumer (DTC) testing (18%), and stem cells and regenerative medicine (5%) (Plunkett-Rondeau et al. 2015). There is little information on teaching integrative medicine, which is very important to patients, since over 40% of the American population already use some type of integrative medicine therapies (Barnes et al. 2008). However, in 2003, 98 out of 126 U.S. medical schools had some teaching of complementary and alternative medicine in their curricula, although most were electives rather than required courses (Starfield et al. 2005). Interestingly, family medicine specialties have been the most receptive of residencies in exploring new strategies for teaching trainees about integrative medicine, perhaps because of family medicine's approach towards "whole-person" health and well-being, including biopsychosocial factors.

The majority of all teaching in medical schools is performed by basic science faculty with PhDs. Therefore, genomics curricula must also be available to graduate students in their PhD programs so that they can keep up to date with the new advances in science and their applications to medicine. Along with genomics courses, a necessary requirement is bioinformatics courses that will cover computer science and programs for studying genomics, proteomics, and epigenetics and for developing algorithms for analyzing large databases.

It is hoped that the pitfalls in simply analyzing a patient's genes for mutations or for diseases are presented to doctors-in-training. Previously, in the discussion on single-nucleotide polymorphisms and genome-wide association study, it is apparent that the genomic approach has not led to the identification of specific genes that are responsible for chronic diseases, such as diabetes and osteoporosis. We know that epigenetics can modify the expression of a gene so that even twins with identical genes can be entirely different in their expression of a particular disease for which they both have the relevant gene. In a *New York Times* article of September 23, 2014 (Grady and Pollack 2014), the story of Tamika Mathews was highlighted. Her grandmother had died young from breast cancer, so she decided to be tested for mutations in two genes that are known to increase the risk for the disease. When a genetics counselor suggested that she be tested for 20 other genes known to be linked to other cancers, she agreed. When the results came to her, she was shocked. She did not have the breast cancer genes, but she did have a mutation in a gene that was linked to stomach cancer. In fact, the mutation is considered so risky that patients are advised to have their stomachs removed. Jennifer was a healthy 39-year-old woman with no family history of stomach cancer, so what should she and her doctors do? Thus, teaching genomics to up-and-coming physicians or already-established physicians seeking to continue their education or wanting to become familiar with the latest in medicine will require us to be cognizant of all of the benefits and the issues in genomics and genetic testing.

NATIONAL RESOURCES FOR GENOMICS TRAINING

With the ability of patients to directly sequence their genomes or have their DNA screened for particular diseases or cancers (DTC genetic testing), patients will soon expect their primary physician to be able to understand and interpret the results of these tests. Several organizations have recently been developed that are entirely or partly dedicated to professional medical education in genetics: the Association of Professors of Human and Medical Genetics (APHMG; http://www.aphmg.org), the American College of Medical Genetics and Genomics (ACMG; http://www.acmg.net), the American Society of Human Genetics (ASHG; http://www.ashg.org), and the National Coalition for Health Professional Education in Genetics (NCHPEG; http://www.nchpeg.org) (Demmer and Waggoner 2014). In addition, the American Board of Medical Genetics has been certifying physicians in clinical genetics since 1982 and has become a member of the American Board of Medical Specialties.

What additional issues need to be addressed with a genomics-based approach to medicine? Even though large-scale sequencing of individual patients is available commercially, there is a lack of databases linking sequence variants with phenotype or disease expression. Even when mutations are found, the data on how many patients will express the mutation and to what extent are not known. When dealing with genetic diseases, counseling of patients and their family members also needs to be considered and implemented. Recently, the Genetics in Primary Care Institute (GPCI; http//www.geneticsinprimarycare.org) was formed through a cooperative agreement between the Health Resources Services Administration, the Maternal and Child Health Bureau, and the American Academy of Pediatrics. Their goal is to provide primary care physicians with the knowledge and skills to address some of the issues in genetics and genomics-based services, especially emphasizing maternal and child health. Another approach for advancing genomics-based medicine is the development of electronic medical records in which specific information and warnings on drugs, genetics risks, and gene–gene and gene–environment interactions can be posted. Other issues that affect the acceptance of genomic medicine include regulatory and reimbursement problems, which are critical for doctors to understand so that their private and hospital practices are solvent.

COLLABORATION ACROSS MEDICAL DISCIPLINES FOR PERSONALIZED MEDICINE

A requirement for implementing personalized medicine is that different doctors from many disciplines work together in order to provide therapies for an individual. Medicine is dominated by specialties: orthopedics, dermatology, neurology, etc. If patients go to different private practices and hospitals for their treatments, then who coordinates all of this information on their personal health? This is a particular issue when medication is prescribed by different physicians. Who is assessing the possible drug interactions and different side effects from medications? Working at a medical center, I have my internist coordinate my medical care, since all of my medical procedures and appointments are at one place. In the computer for each medical specialty are all of my records, which are easily accessible by the physicians at my institution. However, I am lucky to have this great care. Many of my colleagues and friends are on many medications and are seen by physicians at different places. How is their care being coordinated?

Clinical medicine, public health, genetics, statistics, medical sociology, biomedical engineering, molecular biology, and molecular epidemiology need to collaborate in order to provide the best therapy for each individual. Therefore, this requires that most advanced degree programs include personalized medicine in the curriculum of many different specialties in residencies (Lee 2013; Narimatsu et al. 2013). The development of the necessary scientific evidence base that can support clinical practice requires that clinicians and researchers work together with mutual respect for each other's professions, which is not the rule in most hospitals and academic institutions. Teaching physicians to respect other specialties and PhD doctors in science should be a priority, but this topic is never covered in medical school or in residencies. Clinical bioinformatics will have to be developed and easily accessed and understood by physicians who want to practice personalized medicine. There is a need for national bioinformatics programs because, at present, different medical institutions and practices have different computer programs for medical data and they are not compatible with each other. Different databases can prevent physicians from sharing medical information on a patient.

Other issues, such as the ethics of releasing genetic information on individuals, confidentiality, or the ethical/legal dilemma for physicians who are faced with a case in which a patient has a mutation predisposing them to a particular disease, need to be addressed. What information and advice should be given? How can genomic medicine be understood and accepted by the medical community? All of these issues will have to be dealt with in our society. Answers to these questions are uncharted waters in many cases. Personalized medicine will change the paradigm of medical treatment and education from one that is reactive to a medical system that is predictive and preventable, but at what cost?

REFERENCES

Barnes, PM, B Bloom, and RL Nahin. 2008. Complementary and alternative medicine use among adults and children: United States, 2007. *Natl Health Stat Report* (12):1–23.

Demmer, LA and DJ Waggoner. 2014. Professional medical education and genomics. *Annu Rev Genomics Hum Genet* 15:507–16.

Dhar, SU, RL Alford, EA Nelson, and L Potocki. 2012. Enhancing exposure to genetics and genomics through an innovative medical school curriculum. *Genet Med* 14(1):163–7.

Grady, D and A Pollack. 2014. Finding risks, not answers, in gene tests. *New York Times,* September 23, 2014.

LaChance, A and MJ Murphy. 2014. Keeping up with the times: Revising the dermatology residency curriculum in the era of molecular diagnostics and personalized medicine. *Int J Dermatol* 53(11):1377–82.

Lee, RC. 2013. Convolving engineering and medical pedagogies for training of tomorrow's health care professionals. *IEEE Trans Biomed Eng* 60(3):599–601.

Narimatsu, H, C Kitanaka, I Kubota, S Sato, Y Ueno, T Kato, A Fukao, H Yamashita, T Kayama, Yamagata University Medical Education and Training Program through the Genomic Cohort Study. 2013. New developments in medical education for the realization of next-generation personalized medicine: Concept and design of a medical education and training program through the genomic cohort study. *J Hum Genet* 58(9):639–40.

Plunkett-Rondeau, J, K Hyland, and S Dasgupta. 2015. Training future physicians in the era of genomic medicine: Trends in undergraduate medical genetics education. *Genet Med* 17(11):927–31.

Starfield, B, L Shi, and J Macinko. 2005. Contribution of primary care to health systems and health. *Milbank Q* 83:457–502.

10

Drug, hospital, and medical care costs

Can we afford personalized medicine when the U.S. medical care system is the second most expensive medical system in the world?

Discussion on the state of the medical care system in the United States is based on reports from the U.S. Centers for Disease Control and Prevention (CDC) (Figure 10.1). The CDC was begun in 1946 in order to prevent the spread of malaria in the United States. Since 1946, the role of the CDC has expanded and it is now one of the main operating components of the Department of Health and Human Services. The CDC promotes health with agencies prepared to prevent and curtail the spread of disease. When we look at the CDC reports on medical care in the United States that are highlighted in this chapter (National Center for Health Statistics 2014), there are some promising changes occurring in our country's medical care system. Examples that are promising are the decrease in the infant mortality rate, the decrease in infant birth rates in teenagers, the decreases in deaths from heart disease and cancer, and the increases in life expectancy in both males and females to an average of 78.7 years in 2010. In addition, the difference in life expectancy between blacks and whites is narrowing to 3.8 years, but the mortality rate of infants of black mothers is still high at 11.63% compared to 5.20% for whites, but it is decreasing. In 2010, 24% of deaths in the United States were from heart disease and 23% from cancer.

The alarming trends are increases in obesity in adults to 20.4% in 2010. Figure 10.2 shows CDC obesity data from all of the states and territories of the United States, and the alarming rate of obesity in the United States can be clearly seen. As was previously discussed, obesity leads to metabolic syndrome with increased blood pressure, high blood sugar, excess fat around the waist, and abnormal cholesterol levels, leading to an increased risk of diabetes, heart disease, and stroke. Our children under the age of 18 years are also suffering, with 20.5% of children aged 12–19 being obese (in children under 5 years old, obesity has decreased), 5.5% with asthma, 5.2% with food allergies, 9.9% with attention deficit disorder, and 5.8% with serious emotional or behavioral difficulties. In general, personal healthcare expenditure in the United States totaled

Data and Statistics by Topic

- Alcohol use
- Arthritis
- Asthma
- Autism spectrum disorder (ASD)
- Birth defects
- Births and natality
- Blood disorders
- Breastfeeding
- Cancer
- Chronic diseases
- Chronic kidney disease
- Deaths and mortality
- Diabetes
- Foodborne illness
- Genomics
- Heart disease
- Healthy aging
- HIV/AIDS
- Immunizations
- Injuries and violence (Web-Based Injury Statistics Query and Reporting System, WISQARS)
- Life expectancy
- Lyme disease
- Oral health
- Overweight and obesity
- Physical activity
- Reproductive health
- Smoking and tobacco
- Sexually transmitted diseases (STDs)
- Tuberculosis (TB)
- Viral hepatitis

Tools and Resources

- Data.CDC.gov
- CDC Growth Charts
- CDC Vital Signs
- Classification of Diseases, Functioning, and Disability
- Community Health Status Indicators (CHSI 2015)
- Disability and Health Data System
- Health Data Interactive
- Health Indicators Warehouse
- Healthy People 2020
- Interactive Database Tools
- National Program of Cancer Registries
- National Center for HIV/AIDS, Viral Hepatitis, STD, and TB Prevention's (NCHHSTP) Atlas
- The National Institute for Occupational Safety and Health (NIOSH) Data and Statistics Gateway
- Sortable Risk Factors and Health Indicators
- State and Territorial Data
- Surveillance Resource Center
- Surveys and Data Collection Systems
- Vital Stats

Figure 10.1 The Centers for Disease Control and Prevention (CDC). The CDC acquires data and produces statistics on numerous diseases in the United States. It also provides numerous tools and resources for public use, such as on the state of the U.S. medical system broken down by state, health indicators, and growth charts, etc. (Data from CDC website, http://www.cdc.gov/DataStatistics/. Accessed on June 22, 2015.)

$2.3 trillion, according to the CDC, which is an increase of 4.1% from 2010 to 2011, and there are reports that it is as high as $3 trillion now. The average per capita healthcare expenditure was $9255 in 2013.

What will personalized medicine do to per capita healthcare expenditure? There are no data on the effect of personalized medicine costs. However, many of these new personalized therapies are very expensive, since they are targeted at small groups of patients and even individuals. We can find promising changes in costs, such as the sequencing of a human genome, which was discussed in Chapter 3. The sequencing of the first human genome required about $2.7 million, and now the cost has dropped to approximately $1500 per person. However, additional costs, such as analyzing and determining your risk of a disease, add more to the

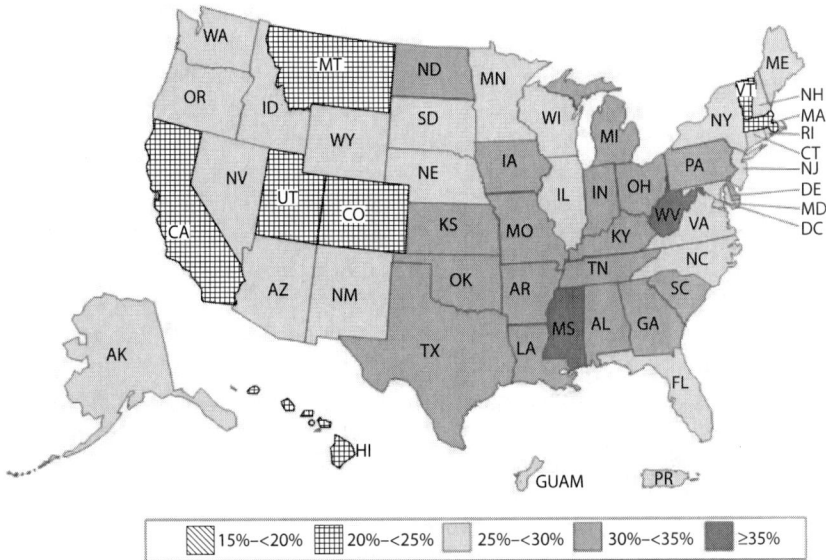

Figure 10.2 Prevalence of obesity among U.S. adults by state and territory in 2013. No state had less than 20% obesity. Seven states and the District of Columbia had between 20% and 25% obesity, while 23 states had a prevalence of obesity of between 25% and 30%. Two states—Mississippi and West Virginia—had rates of 35% or greater. The South had the highest prevalence of obesity (30.2%), followed by the Midwest (30.1%), the Northeast (26.5%), and the West (24.9%). The source of this information came from the Behavioral Risk Factor Surveillance Systems of the CDC.

total price of genetic testing. We also know that factors in epigenetics can modify the expression of particular genes so you cannot be sure that you will ever express the gene that predisposes you to a disease. However, the ability of scientists and companies to find ways to reduce costs is possible, if they are encouraged to do so.

HEALTHCARE COSTS

A promising trend in the medical world is that healthcare costs have slowed substantially in every high-income nation, including the United States, Canada, Britain, France, Germany, and Switzerland, according to the Organization of Economic Cooperation and Development (Mossialos et al. 2015). Explanations specific to one country, such as the enactment of the Affordable Care Act in the United States, cannot explain the changes in all of these countries. However, certain features of the Affordable Care Act are helpful for reducing medical care costs here in the United States. There is increased medical coverage for more people, but a cutback on spending in Medicare has reduced medical care costs, which is mainly due to lower reimbursements to hospitals and insurers. There are also provisions to make the medical care system more efficient by reducing procedures/care that do not make people healthier. We saw this is in the example of the implantable cardioverter–defibrillator (ICD) therapy studies discussed in Chapter 8. ICD was not appropriate for all patients with heart disease, and age and type of heart disease needed to be considered. To address some of these issues, the Affordable Care Act also enacted a board of experts that will consider whether treatments are effective, as this approach has been successful in keeping down costs in European countries.

However, the real reason behind the global slowdown in healthcare expenses may be the economic crisis, which led employers at state, federal, and private levels to provide less generous health insurance plans and to increase out-of-pocket costs for their employees. The economic downturn drove down demands for elective procedures and prevented people who had lost their jobs and medical coverage from seeking medical care. Between 2002 and 2012, in adults aged 18–64, 18.3% had delayed seeking medical care due to cost in the past 12 months compared to 9.7% in 2002 (National Center for Health Statistics 2014). For 9.4% of the adults aged 18–64, prescription drugs were also unattainable due to cost, and this percentage is up from 7.6% in 2002 and continuing to rise. Similar trends are seen in dental care, rising from 10.4% in 2002 to 14.8% in 2012 of the population being unable to take care of their teeth. Other medical care trends are the increase in outpatient care and the decrease in expensive hospital stays. Hospital spending increased 4.3% in 2013 from 2012 levels to $936.9 billion. The increase in hospital spending was less, but it was still considerable. Medicare spending decreased from 2012 to 2103, while Medicaid spending grew 6.1%, an acceleration of 4% compared to 2012, while private health insurance premiums had a lower cost increase in 2013 compared to 2012. The Affordable Care Act is probably responsible for the increase in Medicaid spending, but also the decrease in the rate of hospital spending by the government.

Finally, the global market in pharmaceuticals and devices has increased the use of some of the most efficient drugs and technologies, which has reduced medical costs. For example, the availability of the FibroScan, a less invasive procedure for detecting liver cirrhosis than liver biopsies, is reducing costs. The FibroScan was used in Europe, originating in France from government-sponsored research, and is just now becoming accepted in the United States. It is not invasive and only requires a device to be placed on the skin in order to visualize the liver. The FibroScan uses transient elastography, which is a form of ultrasound, but it is similar in principle to seismology. Liver biopsies can determine whether viruses are affecting the liver, whereas the FibroScan can only test stiffness and steatosis (fatty degeneration), but it measures about 200 times more liver volume than a biopsy. Additional tests such as blood tests can help to determine a viral infection. Finally, some of the patents for popular and common drugs such as Lipitor, a cholesterol drug, and Ambien, a sleeping pill, have expired, and generic drugs for these compounds have significantly brought the prices down for these types of drugs.

DRUG COSTS

On the other hand, pharmaceutical companies have recently increased the prices for some generic drugs, mainly to increase profit. In general, prescription drug expenses totaled $263 billion in 2011, a 2.9% increase from 2010 (National Center for Health Statistics 2014). Retail prescription drug spending grew 2.5% to $27.1 billion, compared to a 0.5% growth in 2012. According to the Intercontinental Marketing Services Health, 84% of all prescriptions were dispensed as generics in 2012. Durable medical equipment, such as contact lenses, eyeglasses, and hearing aids, increased at a slower rate in 2013 compared to 2012, but other non-durable medical products, such as over-the-counter medications, medical instruments, and surgical dressings, grew by 4.0% more to $55.9 billion in 2013.

The United States pays the highest costs for drugs in the world, even compared to other rich nations, such as Canada, Germany, and Japan. The difference in price can often be substantial, especially among the drugs that have just recently come on the market. For example, of the 12 drugs approved by the Food and Drug Administration (FDA) for different cancer indications in 2012, 11 cost more than $100,000 per year. The prices for oncology agents have nearly doubled in the past decade, from an average of $5,000 per month to more than $10,000 per month (Experts in Chronic Myeloid Leukemia 2013). One of the reasons for this is the increase in drugs that are for smaller groups of patients (i.e., more personalized). There are no multiple sclerosis drugs in the United States with a list price of less than $50,000 per year, which is two to three times more than the list price in Canada, Australia, or Britain. In February, Valeant Pharmaceuticals International, Inc., based in Canada, bought the rights to two lifesaving heart drugs, Isuprel and Nitropress, and on the same day, these drug prices rose 525% and 212%, respectively. One vial of Isuprel, used to treat abnormal heart rhythms, rose from $215 to $1347 (Rockoff and Silverman 2015), and for Nitropress from $258 to $806. In response to high drug prices, some states have introduced bills requiring drug makers to report profits and expenses for costly drugs. However, the pharmaceutical companies have helped to defeat such a bill in Oregon, and are presently trying to do the same in California for a bill that would impose reporting requirements on makers of prescription drugs whose wholesale costs are $10,000 or more annually, or per course of treatment.

Another example of increased prescription drug costs is digoxin, used to treat primarily older patients with rapid heart rhythm disturbances (arrhythmias), and was first described in the medical literature in 1785. Three companies selling the drug in the United States have nearly doubled the price they are charging pharmacies since last year, according to EvaluatePharma, a London-based consulting firm (Rosenthal 2014). For patients, this meant that prices at the pharmacy nearly tripled. Remember that many of these older folks are on fixed incomes. One doctor noted that one of his patients was unable to afford her prescription because it would have cost her $1.60 per pill. She did not take her medication and ended up in intensive care. For many patients, there is no effective substitute for digoxin. The World Health Organization has listed digoxin as an essential medicine for the globe. The FDA has stated that there was no drug shortage that might explain this increase in price. The same huge increases in price were being seen for some vaccines for young patients. Other examples of soaring prices for common drugs are codeine, Synthroid, and prednisolone. The percentage of the population taking at least one prescription drug during the past month increased from 39.1% in 1988–1994 to 47.5% in 2007–2010. The percentage of the population taking three or more prescription drugs increased from 11.8% to 20.8%, and those taking more than five drugs more than doubled from 4.0% to 10.1%.

We all need to examine the marketing of drugs and profit motives. Why are drugs pushed on us through our television, which is an expensive place to advertise, when it is your doctor who should be determining what is best for our health? Why would you want to market a particular color of pill without telling you its benefit, which was the case in a recent television advertisement? It appears that drug advertisements are the most pervasive of any type of television advertisement, especially at primetime, maybe only second to advertisements for upcoming programs on that particular network. Why should we take all of these medications unless we really need them, since most, if not all, medications have serious side effects with long-term use? Are there other alternatives to promoting good health rather than pharmaceuticals?

Interestingly, the drugs that are most promoted to doctors by pharmaceutical companies are not medical breakthroughs or cures, but rather are newer drugs. Eliquis, the anticoagulant jointly marketed by Bristol-Myers Squibb and Pfizer, was ranked second (according to the database Open Payments) to the number one drug Victoza from Novo Nordisk, a diabetes medication that also causes an increased risk for thyroid cancer and pancreatitis. Eliquis is an anticoagulant for which the pharmaceutical companies have spent nearly $8 million on marketing to physicians, and has the same benefits as the cheaper drug Coumadin. Its main advantage is that it does not require as much monitoring of the patient's blood.

We also have a conundrum, as evidenced by a recent controversy over the drug Xeljanz for arthritis. Research on this drug was started in a taxpayer-financed laboratory at the National Institutes of Health (NIH), and at that time in 1994, the price of any resulting drug from NIH-financed research had to reflect taxpayer investment. In the next year, the NIH removed this stipulation and Pfizer invested in order to further develop the drug. In 2013, the drug Xeljanz hit the market at a price of $2,055 a month wholesale or $24,666 a year in direct cost to Medicare, without any decrease in the cost due to it being developed first at the NIH. This issue is still being debated and the solution is not clear for pricing and scientific investments (Weisman 2013).

Every month, the CDC identifies a major public health issue. In July 2013, the CDC focused on the rise of prescription painkiller overdoses. Although men are more likely to die from prescription painkiller overdoses than women, the United States has seen this gap closing, with higher rates of overdose in women than have ever seen before. As far as the CDC experts can tell, there is no significant increase in severe pain cases to warrant this increase in painkiller overdoses. Theories on why women are using more prescription painkillers and overdosing is that they suffer more than men with chronic pain and are more likely to be prescribed equivalent or higher doses than men, even though most women have a lower body mass than men. Women are more likely to remain on painkillers than men, and even "shop around" for doctors who will prescribe them. For moderate pain, physical therapy may be a better choice as it can help alleviate the pain, and this approach should be what is first recommended by physicians for patients with moderate pain levels.

WHAT AILS US

When we look at the statistics on what diseases most afflict our global population, we find mental and behavioral disorders at 23.3%, then musculoskeletal disorders at 21.3%, followed by all communicable diseases at 15.5%, and other non-communicable diseases at 11.3% (March et al. 2014) (Figure 10.3). Smaller percentages of chronic respiratory diseases, neurological disorders, injuries, cardiovascular diseases, and cancers afflict the general population. When it comes to musculoskeletal disease, between 5.4% and 12.6% of health expenditure is attributable to musculoskeletal disorders in the world, with 10%–18% of primary care consultation related to this issue. These figures are highest in the United States compared to other countries and regions of the world. Low back pain, neck pain, and osteoarthritis—in descending order of prevalence—are the major issues that contribute to the most years lived with disability.

When we look historically at mental health in the United States, insurance companies have less extensive care for mental health than physical health conditions (Goodell 2014). Patients and their family members are beset with different prior authorization requirements that change every few years, higher cost sharing for patients, and limits on inpatient and outpatient visits. There are so many out-of-pocket expenses for the families of those with mental health conditions that it seems that you have to be rich to obtain consistent and good mental

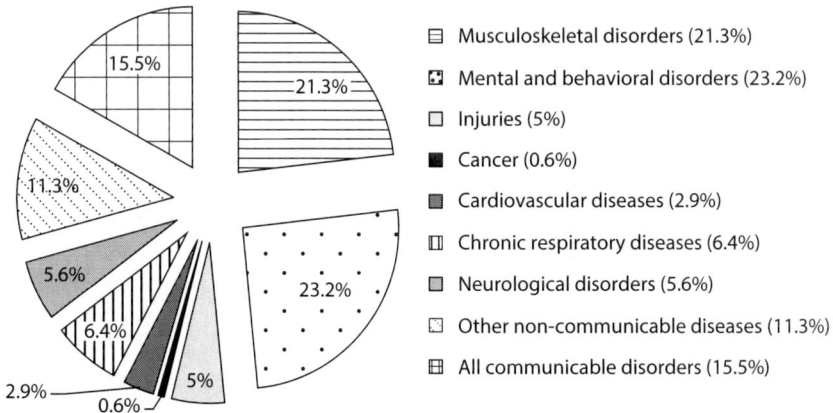

Figure 10.3 A pie chart of diseases that affect our global population. The proportion of different diseases that burden our global population is shown and is based on calculations from data extracted from http://www.healthdata.org/results/data-visualizations in August 2014. The pie chart demonstrates that mental and behavioral disorders are the greatest health burdens in the world, followed by musculoskeletal disorders. (Data from March, L et al. 2014. *Best Pract Res Clin Rheum* 28:353–66.)

healthcare. If you have a family member with mental health issues and deal with this issue, then you understand the predicament. It is not unexpected that we have increased violence from individuals who have fallen through the cracks of our medical system when it comes to mental health. How can we talk about personalized medicine if we do not include and deal appropriately with the major and most prominent health issue(s) of mental health?

Another issue in the United States is excessive alcohol and binge drinking. In a 2011 report from the CDC (CDC 2011), the cost of excessive alcohol consumption in 2006 reached $223.5 billion, at a cost of $746 per person. Approximately 75% of these costs were from binge drinking: consuming four or more alcoholic beverages per occasion for women or five or more drinks at a time for men. Excessive alcohol consumption, or heavy drinking, is defined as consuming an average of more than one alcoholic beverage per day for women or an average of more than two alcoholic beverages per day for men, and any drinking by pregnant women or underage youth. Although this definition of excessive drinking may seem too conservative for those people that drink alcohol, alcohol consumption greater than these guidelines is now known to cause health problems for men and women. Over time, excessive alcohol use can lead to the development of chronic diseases and other serious problems, including cancer, high blood pressure, heart disease, stroke, liver disease, digestive problems, learning and memory problems, and mental health issues, including depression and anxiety. Furthermore, excessive drinking was responsible for 1 in 10 deaths among working-age adults aged 20–64 years. Most of the costs resulted from losses in workplace productivity (72% of total cost), healthcare expenses (11% of cost), law enforcement and criminal justice expenses resulting from excessive alcohol consumption (9% of cost), and motor vehicle crash costs from impaired driving (6% of cost). The study did not consider a number of other costs, such as those due to pain and suffering of the excessive drinker or others who were affected by the drinking, and thus may be an underestimate.

ADDING PERSONALIZED AND PREVENTATIVE MEDICINE TO OUR HEALTHCARE SYSTEM

Although there is no discussion as yet on how personalized medicine will affect the cost of our healthcare system, it is only logical to think that the development of drugs for a small group of patients or individual patients will increase costs. How is our overburdened healthcare system going to deal with this issue? Then there are the other new therapies coming down the pipeline, such as the use of stem cells in regenerative medicine or the sequencing and analysis of individual genomes leading to recommendations on health management that will affect medical treatment for life.

One issue we have is that our healthcare payment system is reversed, in that there are high rewards for expensive procedures and specialties, but not primary and preventative care. Primary and preventative care is practiced most by primary care physicians. The United States has a shortage of primary care physicians that is continuing to grow. By 2035, more than 44,000 primary care physicians will be needed and a shortage of 33,000 is predicted unless 1,700 primary care residency slots are added to the current numbers, or an increase of 21% (Petterson et al. 2015). In 2011, there were 26.1 physicians of all types in patient care per 10,000 people in the United States, ranging from 17.1 in Idaho to 41.1 in Massachusetts and 68.3 in the District of Columbia (National Center for Health Statistics 2014). Thus, we also have a maldistribution of physicians.

To increase the efficiency of our healthcare system, reimbursement to physicians and hospitals is beginning to be tied to outcomes of medical treatments, rather than the expense of procedures and tests. This seems to be opposite to what personalized medicine will bring to the table unless more creative and expense-conscious efforts are made in order to personalize medicine so as to improve patients' health.

The prevailing thought among most doctors is that adding more preventative care to our healthcare system will eventually pay off in reduced healthcare costs. A short description of some of these preventative measures is provided below, and many can be helpful if incorporated into our lifestyles, especially changes in food and drink and increased exercise programs, as discussed in Chapter 4.

Smoking is still a habit that contributes greatly to disease and healthcare costs. As a country, we are reducing the numbers of smokers, but they are still high. According to the CDC, 18.1% of adults aged 18 and over were current cigarette smokers, which is a decline from 23.2% in 2000 (National Center for Health Statistics 2014). Let us be relentless in dealing with the addiction to smoking, help people to stop, and reduce access to tobacco even more, especially for our young people.

Since cigarettes have been discouraged there has been a resurgence of smoking, but the type has changed to e-cigarettes. Many young people are "vaping," the term for using e-cigarettes. E-cigarettes have a battery, a heating element, and a cartridge that holds nicotine and other ingredients, such as flavors. Some are disposable and others have a rechargeable battery and refillable cartridges. Although it is believed that e-cigarettes are less harmful than cigarettes, they are just now being investigated for their health effects. However, e-cigarettes have nicotine inside their cartridges, and nicotine is addictive. Nicotine is dangerous for people with heart conditions and will also harm the arteries over time. Another issue that is still not resolved is the health risk of secondhand smoke from e-cigarettes. A recent study conducted at the Johns Hopkins Bloomberg School of Public Health has shown that exposing mice to e-cigarette vapor resulted in a compromised immune system in the lungs, as well as exposure to potentially dangerous chemicals.

In 2012, 89%–90% of children had completed their childhood vaccinations for diphtheria, tetanus, pertussis, polio, measles, mumps, and rubella (National Center for Health Statistics 2014). Let us make sure that these vaccinations are reasonably priced for everyone. Let us concentrate on clearly explaining to parents the science and rationale behind such important vaccinations for their children in order to prevent these diseases. Let us make sure that these vaccinations are safe, with scientific evidence to allay parents' fears for their children. Let our people become educated in reading and understanding science so that they can make the best decisions for themselves and their families. Writing this book is my attempt as a scientist to address this problem of a lack of communication between doctors and the public. Increasing vaccinations for influenza is also important to prevent pandemics in this country. Vaccinations for pneumococcal and other life-threatening diseases for adults over 65 years of age are also recommended. For adults, at least a yearly visit to the doctor should be required. In 2012, 15.7% of persons had no healthcare visits in the past year, 47.3% had one to three healthcare visits, and 13.1% had 10 or more visits.

Patients are willing to pay out of pocket for preventative care, as can be seen in the use of complementary and alternative medicine (CAM) therapies. In the most comprehensive study to date, approximately 40% of the U.S. population used CAM therapies in 2007, with the most common being natural products that were not minerals or vitamins (Barnes et al. 2008). Many Americans seek CAM therapies for their personal well-being. Other individuals have a medical reason for choosing CAM therapies as they cannot use a particular pharmaceutical product for their condition, have a stress-related disease or a medical condition for which their present allopathic care has not been sufficient or would produce unwanted side effects, or cannot routinely ingest painkillers, etc.

Integrative medicine includes complementary therapies for which there is significant scientific evidence and promotes the relationship between practitioner and patient. Integrative medicine focuses on evidence-based therapies for the individual person and has become a part of personalized medicine. Therefore, it is important to the U.S. population and the medical profession that we determine any efficacy of particular integrative medicine/complementary therapies. The majority of cancer patients have been shown to use some type of CAM therapy (Garland et al. 2013; Deng and Cassileth 2014; Huebner et al. 2014). Out-of-pocket expenses that included CAM therapies accounted for 12% of national health spending, growing by 3.2% in 2013 to $339.4 billion. In 2013, households accounted for the largest share of spending (28%) on CAM therapies, followed by the federal government at 26%, private businesses at 21%, and state and local government at 17%. The U.S. population is willing to become engaged in helping themselves heal and should be encouraged to do so, but it is also important to know what CAM therapies have the ability to improve health. In addition, more medical insurance companies should provide reimbursement for CAM therapies that are beneficial for their patients. Most CAM therapies are not reimbursed and CAM practitioners have to volunteer their services at hospitals to help patients.

Doctors die differently. The *Wall Street Journal*, the *Journal of Medicine*, and other medical journals featured articles by Ken Murray, MD. The opening paragraph of the article reads as follows:

"Years ago, Charlie, a highly respected orthopedist and a mentor of mine, found a lump in his stomach. It was diagnosed as pancreatic cancer by one of the best surgeons in the country, who had developed a procedure that could triple a patient's five-year-survival odds—from 5% to 15%—albeit with a poor quality of life. Charlie, 68 years old, was uninterested. He went home the next day, closed his practice and never set foot in a hospital again. He focused on spending time with his family. Several months later, he died at home. He got no chemotherapy, radiation or surgical treatment. Medicare didn't spend much on him."

What appears to be at first a mystery is that doctors go for less treatment than other Americans, especially when it comes to dying. Perhaps they understand best what the medical options are, and choose to make decisions that preserve the quality of their lives at the end. This topic needs to be discussed in every state. People need to be given choices in the most realistic terms and their families and friends need to respect their choices.

The same week that I wrote this section, Canada's Supreme Court ruled that doctors may help patients who have severe and incurable medical conditions to die. This ruling overturns a 1993 ban. The case was brought to the Supreme Court of Canada by a civil rights group representing two women, Kay Carter and Gloria Taylor, with degenerative diseases. Both died before they could hear the outcome of their case. The government now has a year to rewrite its law on assisted suicide or else the current law will be struck down. In Canada, it is illegal to counsel, aid, or abet a suicide, with penalties of up to 14 years in prison. On the other hand, Switzerland allows "assisted suicide" that does not require a terminal illness, but must be performed by the patient and has led to "suicide tourism" across Europe. Canada is not the only place where this issue has come to the forefront.

In the United States, 29-year-old Brittany Maynard, who had a brain tumor, was forced to travel from California, where the practice of assisted suicide is illegal, to Oregon, where it has been legal since 1997. On November 2, 2014, *People* magazine and various other media sources reported that Maynard had ended her life on November 1 surrounded by her loved ones. In accordance with Oregon state law regarding death with dignity, a brain tumor is recorded as the official cause of death on her death certificate. Maynard wrote in her final Facebook post: "Goodbye to all my dear friends and family that I love. Today is the day I have chosen to pass away with dignity in the face of my terminal illness, this terrible brain cancer that has taken so much from me … but would have taken so much more."

There is a profound difference of opinion on the issue of assisted dying, with some believing that it is a fundamental human right versus those who have ethical objections and worry about the implications for the disabled and vulnerable. It is an important debate with no easy answers, but it will need to be resolved and it will have a major effect on our healthcare system (Figure 10.4).

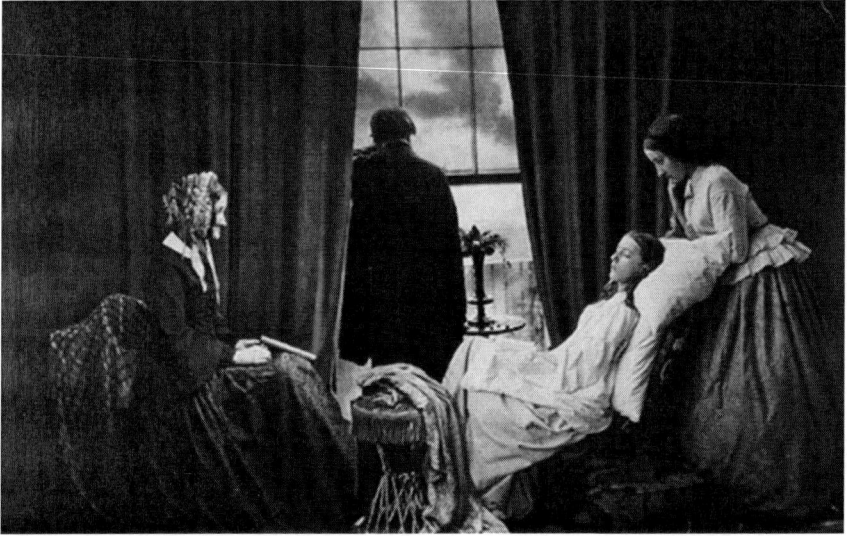

Figure 10.4 A photograph of death and dying from Henry Peach Robinson (1830–1901). This photograph was taken by the English pictorialist photographer and is called "Fading Away" (1858).

CONCLUSIONS

As we move forward in healthcare and as the U.S. population increases in the number of aging individuals, it appears that personalized medicine and healthcare costs are on a collision course. How they will interact to provide us with the best care at the most reasonable price for our country is anyone's guess. As a scientist (my bias), I think that investing in science will lead to new discoveries for improving our healthcare system, but unfortunately we do not know from where these new discoveries will come. Therefore, it is important not only to invest in clinically relevant research, but also in the basic science of our cells and genes, as well as other organisms. Nature has a myriad of solutions for allowing life in different environments. Basic science has yielded many important solutions to disease. For example, it has been estimated that 60% of the drugs that are now available, which include such household names as artemisinin (a derivative that treats malaria), camptothecin (used as an anti-cancer drug to inhibit DNA enzyme topoisomerase I), lovastatin (for cardiovascular disease), paclitaxel (anti-cancer), penicillin, reserpine (an antipsychotic and antihypertensive drug), etc., are either directly or indirectly derived from natural products (Newman 2008).

A major overhaul of our medical care system is also required for us to sustain our medical costs. The three basics—education, health, and international relationships/protection—should be the purview of our government. These three principles are the reasons why governments should exist to create equitable and cost-effective solutions to educating and caring for a country's population. Allowing other types of businesses to flourish independently is also important, but why should profits be made on a person's health misfortune? Our government should also negotiate with pharmaceutical companies to lower the prices on essential medications. Incentives to take better care of ourselves should also be incorporated into our healthcare system. What other role is more important for a government than ensuring the pursuing of these three fundamental human activities and creating a healthy, intellectually engaged, and safe country?

REFERENCES

Barnes, PM, B Bloom, and RL Nahin. 2008. Complementary and alternative medicine use among adults and children: United States, 2007. *Natl Health Stat Report* (12):1–23.

CDC. 2011. *CDC Online Newsroom October 17*. www.cdc.gov/media/releases/2011/p1017_alcohol_consumption.html.

Deng, G and B Cassileth. 2014. Integrative oncology: An overview. *Am Soc Clin Oncol Educ Book* 2014:233–42.

Experts in Chronic Myeloid Leukemia (119 authors). 2013. The price of drugs for chronic myeloid leukemia (CML) is a reflection of the unsustainable prices of cancer drugs: From the perspective of a large group of CML experts. *Blood* 121(22):4439–42.

Garland, SN, D Valentine, K Desai, S Li, C Langer, T Evans, and JJ Mao. 2013. Complementary and alternative medicine use and benefit finding among cancer patients. *J Altern Complement Med* 19(11):876–81.

Goodell, S. 2014. Health policy brief: Mental health parity. *Health Affairs*, April 3, 2014.

Huebner, J, FJ Prott, O Micke, R Muecke, B Senf, G Dennert, K Muenstedt, and PRIO (Working Group Prevention and Integrative Oncology—German Cancer Society). 2014. Online survey of cancer patients on complementary and alternative medicine. *Oncol Res Treat* 37(6):304–8.

March, L, EUR Smith, DG Hoy, MJ Cross, L Sanchez-Riera, F Blyth, R Buchbinder, T Vos, and AD Woolf. 2014. Burden of disability due to musculoskeletal (MSK) disorders. *Best Pract Res Clin Rheum* 28:353–66.

Mossialos, E, M Wenzl, R Osborn, and C Anderson (editors). 2015. *International Profiles of Health Care Systems, 2014*. Australia, Canada, Denmark, England, France, Germany, Italy, Japan, the Netherlands, New Zealand, Norway, Singapore, Sweden, Switzerland, and the United States. The Commonwealth Fund. http://www.commonwealthfund.org/publications/fund-reports/2015/jan/international-profiles-2014.

National Center for Health Statistics. 2014. *Health, United States, 2013. With Special Feature on Prescription Drugs*. Hyattsville, MD: Library of Congress.

Newman, DJ. 2008. Natural products as leads to potential drugs: An old process or the new hope for drug discovery? *J Med Chem* 51:2589–99.

Petterson, SM, WR Liaw, C Tran, and AW Bazemore. 2015. Estimating the residency expansion required to avoid projected primary care physician shortages by 2035. *Ann Family Med* 13(2):107–14.

Rockoff, JD and E Silverman. 2015. Pharmaceutical companies buy rivals' drugs, then jack up the prices. *Wall Street J*, April 26, 2015.

Rosenthal, E. 2014. Rapid price increases for some generic drugs catch users by surprise. *New York Times*, July 9, 2014.

Weisman, J. 2013. Seeking profits for taxpayers in potential of new drug. *New York Times*, March 19, 2013.

11

Ethics

How important is ethics for personalized medicine?

Ethics are an important cornerstone of human civilization and are critical in medicine and research. Recognition of the importance of ethics can be found in the Western world's rite of passage for a new physician who takes the Hippocratic Oath to uphold ethical standards. The Hippocratic Oath is believed to be derived from Hippocrates, the father of Western medicine, and was written in the late fifth century BCE (Figure 11.1). A more modern version is now used in many countries and is presented below. The Hippocratic Oath still rings true today and it describes those qualities most important in medicine: not only to remember the science, but also "that warmth, sympathy, and understanding may outweigh the surgeon's knife or the chemist's drug," to respect the privacy of the patient, and to prevent disease, since prevention is preferable to cure.

Hippocratic Oath (modern version written by Louis Lasagna, Academic Dean of the School of Medicine at Tufts University):

I swear to fulfill, to the best of my ability and judgment, this covenant:

I will respect the hard-won scientific gains of those physicians in whose steps I walk, and gladly share such knowledge as is mine with those who are to follow.

I will apply, for the benefit of the sick, all measures which are required, avoiding those twin traps of overtreatment and therapeutic nihilism.

I will remember that there is art to medicine as well as science, and that warmth, sympathy, and understanding may outweigh the surgeon's knife or the chemist's drug.

I will not be ashamed to say "I know not," nor will I fail to call in my colleagues when the skills of another are needed for a patient's recovery.

I will respect the privacy of my patients, for their problems are not disclosed to me that the world may know. Most especially must I tread with care in matters of life and death. If it is given me to save a life, all thanks. But it may also be within my power to take a life; this awesome

---

responsibility must be faced with great humbleness and awareness of my own frailty. Above all, I must not play at God.

I will remember that I do not treat a fever chart, a cancerous growth, but a sick human being, whose illness may affect the person's family and economic stability. My responsibility includes these related problems, if I am to care adequately for the sick.

I will prevent disease whenever I can, for prevention is preferable to cure.

I will remember that I remain a member of society, with special obligations to all my fellow human beings, those sound of mind and body as well as the infirm.

If I do not violate this oath, may I enjoy life and art, respected while I live and remembered with affection thereafter. May I always act so as to preserve the finest traditions of my calling and may I long experience the joy of healing those who seek my help.

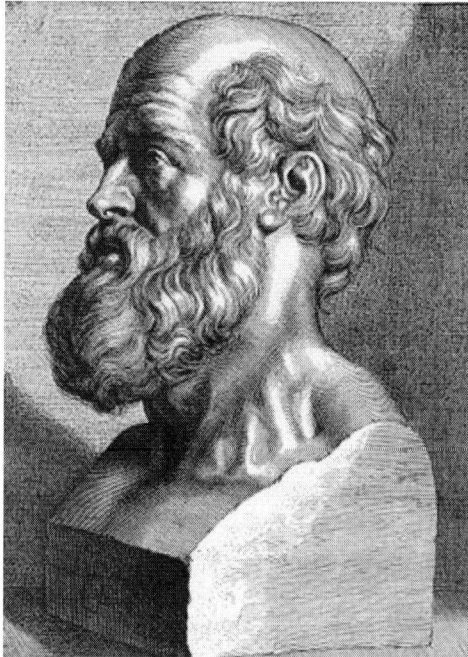

Figure 11.1 Engraving of Hippocrates by Peter Paul Rubens from 1638. Hippocrates was a Greek physician in Classical Greece and is considered the "father of Western medicine" in recognition of his contributions to medicine and as the founder of the Hippocratic School of Medicine. This school revolutionized medicine in ancient Greece and established medicine as its own discipline, rather than being associated with theurgy (the practice of rituals, often considered magical or evoking one or more gods) and philosophy. The Hippocratic Oath is also attributed to Hippocrates.

However, the history of man has shown that this oath was not enough to prevent atrocities such as those committed during war, as in World War II, or from medical experimentation, an example of which is the syphilis testing on African–Americans. In 1932, the Public Health Service, working with the Tuskegee Institute in Tennessee, started a study initially with 600 black men without the benefit of the patients' informed consent. Researchers told the men that they were being treated for "bad blood," a slang term used at that time to describe syphilis, anemia, and fatigue. These men never received the proper treatment needed to treat their illness, but were promised free medical examinations, free meals, and burial insurance. The study lasted for 40 years and was ended in 1972, many years after the 1947 discovery that penicillin could cure them.

LAWS PROTECTING PATIENTS

The world needs laws to protect patients from medical and scientific experimentation. The Nuremberg Code is a set of ethical principles for research on human subjects that was developed as a result of the Nuremberg trials at the end of the Second World War (Figure 11.2). These trials focused on Nazi officials who were involved in killings and also sent people to concentration camps where they were executed, and doctors who performed human experimentation on the people sent to concentration camps. It is believed that over 3,500,000 sterilizations were part of these experiments, and many other types of experiments were performed forcibly on people in concentration camps.

The Nuremberg Code requires that any experimentation needs patient consent without any force or stress to the patient. The patient has the right to terminate any procedure or treatment at any time. No experiment should be unnecessary, and it should have value for the society and be based on previous knowledge. Each experiment should be conducted so as to avoid all unnecessary physical and mental injury or pain. The facilities in which these experiments are performed should be medically adequate in order to prevent any harm, and experiments should be performed by scientifically qualified persons, among other stipulations.

The following ten points are from the U.S. National Institutes of Health "Nuremberg Code," retrieved on June 20, 2012:

1. The voluntary consent of the human subject is absolutely essential. This means that the person involved should have legal capacity to give consent; should be so situated as to be able to exercise free power of choice, without the intervention of any element of force, fraud, deceit, duress, over-reaching, or other ulterior form of constraint or coercion; and should have sufficient knowledge and comprehension of the elements of the subject matter involved as to enable him/her to make an understanding and enlightened

decision. This latter element requires that before the acceptance of an affirmative decision by the experimental subject there should be made known to him the nature, duration, and purpose of the experiment; the method and means by which it is to be conducted; all inconveniences and hazards reasonable to be expected; and the effects upon his health or person which may possibly come from his participation in the experiment. The duty and responsibility for ascertaining the quality of the consent rests upon each individual who initiates, directs or engages in the experiment. It is a personal duty and responsibility which may not be delegated to another with impunity.

2. The experiment should be such as to yield fruitful results for the good of society, unprocurable by other methods or means of study, and not random and unnecessary in nature.

3. The experiment should be so designed and based on the results of animal experimentation and a knowledge of the natural history of the disease or other problem under study that the anticipated results will justify the performance of the experiment.

4. The experiment should be so conducted as to avoid all necessary physical and mental suffering and injury.

5. No experiment should be conducted where there is a prior reason to believe that death or disabling injury will occur; except, perhaps, in those experiments where the experimental physicians also serve as subjects.

6. The degree of risk to be taken should never exceed that determined by the humanitarian importance of the problem to be solved by the experiment.

7. Proper preparations should be made and adequate facilities provided to protect the experimental subject against even remote possibilities of injury, disability, or death.

8. The experiment should be conducted only by scientifically qualified persons. The highest degree of skill and care should be required through all stages of the experiment of those who conduct or engage in the experiment.

9. During the course of the experiment the human subject should be at liberty to bring the experiment to an end if he has reached the physical or mental state where continuation of the experiment seems to him to be impossible.

10. During the course of the experiment the scientist in charge must be prepared to terminate the experiment at any stage, if he has probable cause to believe, in the exercise of the good faith, superior skill and careful judgment required of him that a continuation of the experiment is likely to result in injury, disability, or death to the experimental subject.

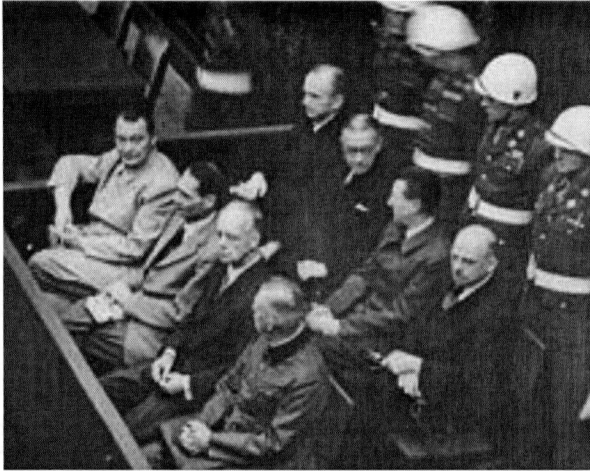

Figure 11.2 An old picture of the Nuremberg trials that investigated the atrocities committed during World War II by the Nazis in Germany. In the dock are seen the defendants (in front row, from left to right): Hermann Göring, Rudolf Heß, Joachim von Ribbentrop, and Wilhelm Keitel; (in second row, from left to right): Karl Dönitz, Erich Raeder, Baldur von Schirach, and Fritz Saukel. The main target of the prosecution was Hermann Göring, considered to be the most important surviving official of the Third Reich after Hitler's death. He was originally the second highest-ranked member of the Nazi Party. He was the Commander of the Luftwaffe from 1935 to 1945, Chief of the Four-Year Plan from 1936 to 1945, and original head of the Gestapo before turning it over to the Schutzstaffel (SS paramilitary group) in 1934. He committed suicide on the night before his execution.

In addition to trying to ensure the ethical behavior of physicians towards their patients, other documents, such as the Declaration of Helsinki, set ethical standards for research and other types of human experimentation. It was developed by the World Medical Association, and although it is not legally binding under international law, it has been accepted and used throughout the world. Since its inception in 1964 in Helsinki, Finland, it has undergone numerous revisions. In 1979, the United States also created the Belmont Report: Ethical Principles and Guidelines for the Protection of Human Subjects of Research, Report of the National Commission for the Protection of Human Subjects of Biomedical and Behavioral Research. The Belmont Report deals with informed consent, assessment of risks and benefits, and selection of subjects for scientific experiments.

When I was in my early teens, my father took a trip to Boston, leaving my mother at home with me since I had to go to school. They were very secretive about the trip. Many years later, I came to find out that my father had visited a very close friend, Sasha, and his wife in Boston, where she was undergoing surgery to try to correct experimental work performed on her in a Nazi concentration camp. We did not see them too often since they owned a chocolate factory in Venezuela, which I would benefit from at holidays with a package from them. They never had children and she was crippled from the experimentation. Sasha never forgot my father's kindness, and years later, after his wife had died, he was the last friend of the family to see my father before he died. So many people were affected by the crimes of World War II, and I did not know until I was older about these and other events in my family, and how this tragic piece of history had affected my family and friends so directly.

PRIVACY OF PATIENT RECORDS AND HIPAA

Impressive advances in genome sequencing and increased understanding of how a particular gene, mutation, or sequence may relate to a disease or respond to treatment bring promising improvements to personalized medicine and preventative care. However, with this progress come new issues of privacy that need to be addressed.

How are we going to protect private medical information when even the National Security Agency (NSA) cannot protect its own secrets? The NSA scandal developed when Edward Snowden, a former system administrator for the Central Intelligence Agency (CIA), worked for the NSA. He disclosed to several media outlets classified documents that revealed numerous global surveillance programs run by the NSA and the Five Eyes with the cooperation of telecommunication companies. The Five Eyes are an intelligence alliance bound by a multilateral UKUSA Agreement, consisting of Australia, Canada, New Zealand, the United Kingdom, and the United States, who have cooperated in signals intelligence since World War II, and this agreement remains in existence to this day. Snowden had expressed concern to his superiors over the broad nature of these surveillance programs, but no one addressed his concerns and inquiries. He took matters into his own hands and released documents on the broad nature of U.S. government surveillance, which he considered unconstitutional, but others have considered them to be a part of national security.

In the Snowden case, our private e-mails and internet inquiries were being given by private companies with whom we have accounts to the government to view, store, and use. I remember the late 1950s and 1960s when wiretaps in general required a court order and to show cause for suspecting someone of wrongdoing, yet were kept secret. There is no justice system oversight for NSA activities, which has raised questions of our national security and what is constitutional when it entails acquiring data on American citizens who have no criminal records or are not under suspicion of wrongdoing. It also brings into question how private information can be protected. Examples of this private information are health records or e-mails about health issues between physicians and/or their staff members and/or insurance company staffers. We do not want any of this information to be used against us in situations such as employment, assessment of health insurance premiums, etc. What if you had hepatitis C or HIV and no one would hire you? What if you discovered you had a collagen disease that made you more susceptible to injuries while you are a physical therapist? You might lose your job or never be promoted. Or what if you had a nervous breakdown 5 years ago, worked for the past 5 years, but your employer closed up shop, and now you are looking for a job? Or what if you simply wanted to have your health information protected from your friends, families, and strangers. You might not want everyone in your family to know that you had experienced a nervous breakdown 5 or 10 years ago. Individuals are susceptible to discrimination due to their present medical conditions and even their past medical conditions. There have been some positive steps towards ensuring the privacy of our health information; however, personalized medicine and the new era of genomics create new problems that require solutions.

A positive step towards protecting patients' personal health records has come from the federal Health Insurance Portability and Accountability Act (HIPAA) of 1996 (Figure 11.3). In medicine, electronic databases of patients' records are protected by the HIPAA. The law makes it easier for healthcare providers to keep health insurance information, control administrative costs involved with

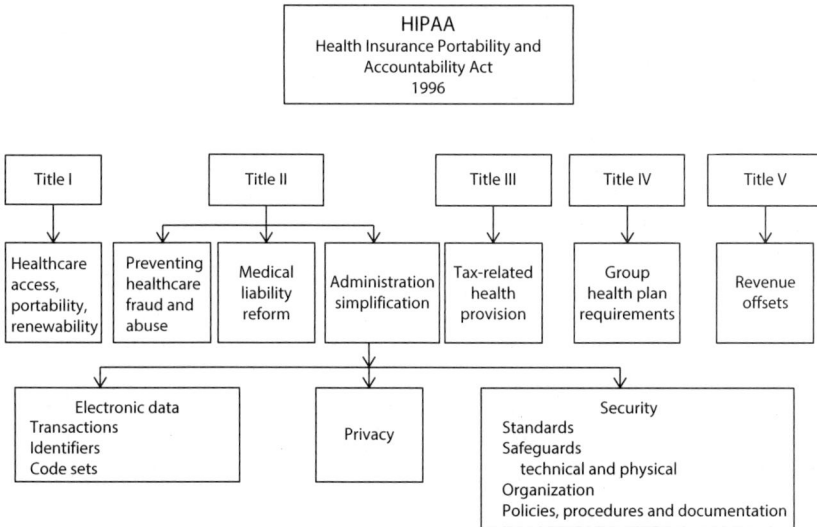

Figure 11.3 The Health Insurance Portability and Accountability Act (HIPAA) that was created in 1996. A brief description of the various titles of the Act is given. Title I of the HIPAA protects health insurance coverage for workers and their families when they change or lose their jobs. Title II of the HIPAA, known as the Administrative Simplification provisions, established national standards for electronic healthcare transactions and national identifiers for providers, health insurance plans, and employers. Title III of the HIPAA standardizes the amount of money that may be saved per person in a pre-tax medical savings account. Title IV of the HIPAA specifies the conditions for group health plans regarding the coverage of persons with pre-existing conditions, and modifies continuation of coverage requirements. Title V of the HIPAA deals with revenue governing tax deductions for employers providing health coverage. It also amends the laws dealing with people who give up U.S. citizenship or permanent residence.

transmitting pertinent information on patients, and protect the confidentiality and security of healthcare information. However, all of this information is electronically based and is susceptible to hacking. When we go to the doctor's office, we often sign the HIPAA forms that describe the confidential nature of our health records and their protection, along with any additional changes in the law.

In the book *Girl in Glass*, Deanna Fei (2015) describes her experiences after giving birth prematurely, while just 5.5 months pregnant. Minutes later, she met her tiny baby, who clung to life inside a glass box. Her daughter spent most of her first year of life in the hospital as she fought for her life. A year after her birth, Fei brought her daughter home from the hospital. At that time, her husband's employer and CEO at America Online (AOL), Tim Armstrong, cut employees' benefits and blamed the need for the cuts on the expense of the birth of Deanna's daughter and another family with a premature baby, whom he did not identify by family name but called "distressed babies." This set off a national firestorm. Mothers' advocates criticized him for gross insensitivity. Lawyers debated whether he had violated his employees' privacy. Healthcare experts noted that blaming "million-dollar babies" for cutting other employees' benefits was unlikely. It also highlighted the issue of the lack of medical privacy that families experience when they are faced with a medical issue that is accessible by their employer. This story surfaced even with the HIPAA regulations in place, and was not covered by the HIPAA. Deanna's daughter, Mila, is now several years old and appears to be perfectly normal. After all of the publicity, Tim Armstrong decided not to implement the cut in employees' benefits and apologized.

Each genome is unique and identifies its owner, and thus it contains highly personal and crucially private data that need to be protected by our society. Therefore, standards are needed for data protection in hospitals and private companies performing genetic screenings.

PATIENT AUTONOMY, WELL-BEING, AND EQUITY

In the narrow view of personalized medicine as tailoring the responses of molecular receptors to achieve the best medical outcomes for a patient, bioethicists have identified several areas in which patients need to be protected: (1) patient autonomy and agency; (2) patient well-being; (3) preventing or minimizing harm; and (4) promoting fairness and equity (Lewis et al. 2014). Protecting autonomy of a patient provides each individual with the right to know or not to know about their predisposition for a disease. No individual, company, or insurance provider should be able to force someone to take a test that would determine whether they have a likelihood of developing a particular disease.

Predictive tests for disease susceptibility in personalized medicine can negatively influence a patient's sense of well-being, which could affect their health. It is important to provide patients and doctors with appropriate tools to counsel patients on medical options and provide additional support for such issues as the effect of knowing life expectancy or the need to make lifestyle changes for better survival.

> In my neighborhood, a local private high school asked students if they wanted to submit to DNA screening as part of their molecular biology class. Letters were sent home to parents to ask permission. My question is: is this ethical? I can imagine some teenagers being eager to find out about their genes. However, what if this screening uncovered a mutation in a gene that might cause a disease? How would the school handle this, or the parents, or the teenager? Who is available in this situation to counsel them? At this point in time, individuals can have DNA screening performed for a fee. Should anyone, anywhere, be able to do this on their own? Is this one's right as an individual? If it is a right, is one receiving appropriate counseling on the impact of that information?

Personalized therapeutic measures may also cause an ethical dilemma leading to unequal access to a particular therapy. For example, an expensive drug may be prescribed for a young person, but if that person was 65 years of age with fewer years to live, would the healthcare system want to spend the money on an expensive therapy? How can patients be treated equally in a personalized medical system? What other distributional issues could develop with personalized medicine? Personalized medicine also proposes to determine whether patients are good responders or poor responders to a particular drug or treatment regimen. With this information, who will decide whether that patient will be allowed to go through with that therapy? Funding the diagnostic test along with the companion treatment that is most likely to succeed would reduce waste and cost in the medical care system. Would some molecularly targeted treatments only be affordable to those wealthy enough to pay for them? Or will companies still develop these treatments for high profit and pass off the costs or cut back on the scientific investigation of more affordable but less profitable therapies?

An example of equity issues in personalized medicine can be seen when the Australian Pharmaceutical Benefits Advisory Committee recommended against including trastuzumab (Herceptin) for national consumption for the treatment of metastatic breast cancer. It was not considered cost effective for the majority of patients. Public and medical outcry pressured the government to set up a special fund outside the national formulary to fund Herceptin treatments (Mackenzie et al. 2008). The United States and other countries, especially poorer countries trying to establish universal healthcare systems, are facing these issues, particularly when it comes to expensive targeted cancer therapies. Weighing the benefits of efficiency with equity in healthcare has ethical ramifications that society will have to consider regardless of the "greater good" for the patient.

PERSONALIZED THERAPEUTICS

In personalized medicine, establishing small patient subgroups for a therapeutic measure may lead to insufficient drug testing before patient application, and could result in higher risks for patients. There may also be increased false-positive prognostic test results that need to be determined and minimized in order to calculate a test's accuracy. In addition, personalized medicine often requires both a diagnostic test for a biomarker of a disease and then a treatment. This makes it more difficult for randomization in a randomized controlled trial to test drug efficacy, and would lead to double randomization in order to evaluate the benefits of a particular treatment. It is difficult to envision how the different arms of this double randomization (taking the diagnostic test or not, being treated or not) would be acceptable to human research ethics committees for evaluating the efficacy of tests and treatments. The use of historical or contemporary biomarker cohorts may be a way to deal with this issue, but this aspect of personalized medicine certainly complicates the interpretation of efficacy and can increase costs of testing.

Many of the drugs developed for personalized medicine are for acute health issues, such as cancer. They are used for only a short period of time, which does not allow pharmaceutical companies to recoup drug discovery costs, compared to the drugs used for more extended periods of times, such as bronchodilators for asthma or lipid-lowering drugs that patients take for the rest of their lives in order to prevent heart disease.

Several studies have suggested that as many as two-thirds of the "disease-causing mutations" found in the Human Genome Database may have low to no clinically meaningful pathogenicity (Dorschner et al. 2015; Wilson and Nicholls 2015). Many gene variants of unknown significance have been found, and there is a lack of understanding of the natural history of risk for well-known gene variants, which makes overdiagnosis and overtreatment prevalent for conditions that may never be manifested in someone's lifetime. It is estimated that a genome screen of an average patient would generate hundreds of false-positive test results.

Once the results of a test have been obtained and it has been determined that a patient has a chance of developing a disease, how do we medically insure patients with a genetic mutation with the potential of being expressed? In the United States, the 2008 Genetic Information Nondiscrimination Act prohibits group health plans and insurers from denying coverage or charging higher premiums to healthy individuals based on genetic test results (Wilson and Nicholls 2015). However, who will police insurers and what are the penalties? At this point, we do not have a system in place that will advocate for patients that are discriminated against, and once a claim is denied, how will the patients be informed of why this denial has occurred? A 2013 systematic review on this topic concluded that there was not good evidence for the prevalence of this type of discriminatory practice (Joly et al. 2013). In some cases, it also appears difficult to distinguish between family history issues versus genetic tests influencing insurance policies. However, we now have the example of *Girl in Glass* and how the employer gained access to private health information and tried to use it to penalize all of the employees in his company.

RESEARCH ETHICS

The ultimate personalized treatment would be to edit genes so that all cells in an organ or in an individual would express the change, which could even be passed on from generation to generation. However, most scientists know that the stem cell biology field is not ready to begin genetically manipulating human embryos. A moratorium on genome editing in human embryos using current technologies has been called for by numerous scientific groups due to our lack of knowledge and techniques at this point in time making this work dangerous, with unpredictable effects and ethically unacceptable outcomes (Guerts et al. 2009; Lanphier et al. 2015).

One of the other concerns from scientists is that the negative impacts of results on embryos might lead to the prohibition of genome-editing techniques, especially on somatic (non-reproductive) cells that do not have the ability to be inherited. This is a slippery slope because any genetic manipulation to repair or eliminate a mutation in a particular tissue of adult humans with this technology might also result in harm or even death. Difficulties arise when private companies, in partnership with private hospitals, seek to "experiment" without public/governmental knowledge and regulation. Fifteen of 22 European nations have prohibited the modification of the germline (Lanphier et al. 2015). This time, the United States has not officially prohibited germline modifications.

Editing of genes in human embryos has been tried in China with disastrous results, as had been predicted (Kolata 2015; Liang et al. 2015). Scientists did not plan to produce a baby, but used 85 defective human embryos from a fertility clinic for their work. Mature oocytes were inseminated and only those that were abnormal with three pronuclei were selected for research. The method for gene editing that was applied was clustered regularly interspersed short palindromic repeats-associated protein 9 (CRISPR/Cas9), a bacteria-derived system that uses RNA to recognize specific human DNA sequences and then uses an endonuclease, Cas9, to cut the required sequence for genetic manipulation. In this case, the β-globin gene was targeted. β-globin is a heme-containing protein involved in binding and transporting oxygen in red blood cells. CRISPR/Cas9 was able to cleave the endogenous β-globin gene, but DNA repair after the cut was low and created mosaics in which some cells had the edited gene and other cells did not. Additional genes besides β-globin were cleaved and other mutations developed. Thus, the experiment had failed, and showed the lack of knowledge regarding using this technology to edit genes successfully. Besides CRISPR/Cas9, there are other techniques, such as the use of zinc-finger nucleases (ZFNs), which are DNA-binding proteins that can be engineered to cause a break in DNA. ZFNs allow scientists to knock out specific genes, repair a mutation, or add new DNA.

These experiments introduce serious ethical questions that need to be addressed by the United States and the scientific community at large, especially in industry. This controversy is not all bad; for example, Sangamo Biosciences is conducting clinical trials to evaluate ZFN-based genome editing for HIV/AIDS (Tebas et al. 2014), with mixed success. More work is needed before this approach would be ready for the general population with HIV/AIDS.

ARTIFICIAL INTELLIGENCE

In the twenty-first century, artificial intelligence is starting to tell doctors how to treat us (Figure 11.4). One of the programs using artificial intelligence is Modernizing Medicine, an iPad electronic medical assistant (EMA) system for various medical specialties. Recently, an example in dermatology was presented (Hernandez 2014). A dermatologist, Dr. Kavita Mariwalla, specializes in acne, burns, and rashes. However, when a patient with a disfiguring case of bullous pemphigoid—a rare skin condition resulting in large watery blisters—entered her office, she was not sure how to treat her, especially since a medication for the auto-immune disorder was not available. She used the Modernizing Medicine website to find a medication for her patient, and was able to help her. This web-based program is available around the country and is supposed to be based on data from doctors and their patients. However, what if this web-based program was wrong? How does a doctor interpret the data on the website to give the best care? Is the website and information peer reviewed like scientific and medical publications, as discussed in Chapter 8? These are just some of the issues facing the medical

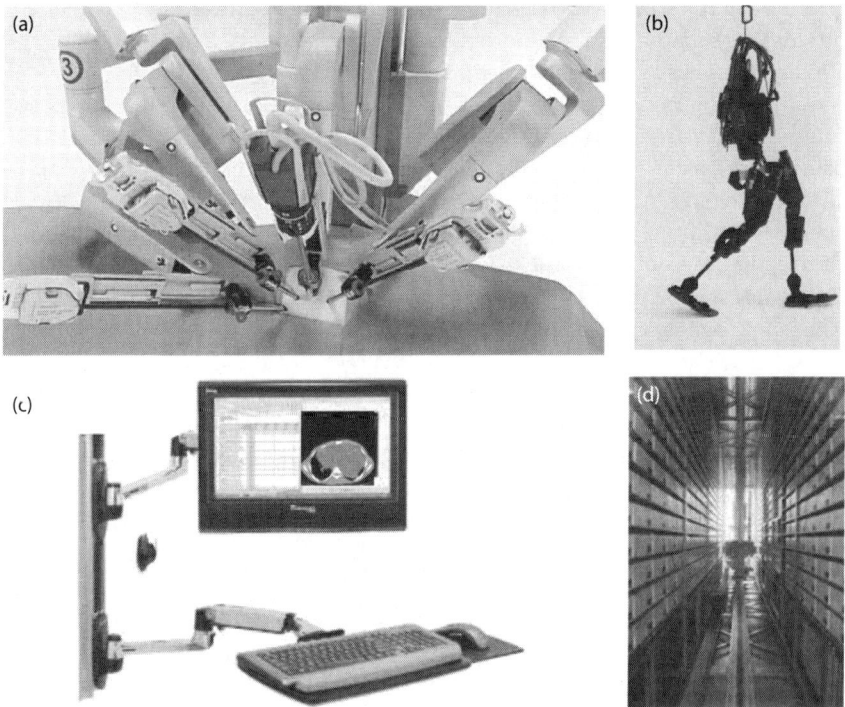

(a)

(b)

(c)

(d)

Figure 11.4 Artificial intelligence. Different types of artificial intelligence in medicine are shown. In (a), simulated robotic surgery is shown. In (b), artificial limbs are illustrated. In (c), computers are shown that deal with medical issues, diagnosis, and treatment, and are often seen in hospitals. In (d), a drug dispensary that is computerized is illustrated.

profession in personalized medicine in the era of artificial intelligence. Yes, the data are based on human knowledge, but how do we know that the conclusions are correct for all patients and for the particular patient in front of us?

Artificial intelligence is in its early stages and cannot match our own intelligence, and computers cannot replace doctors at the bedside. The positive side of artificial intelligence and supercomputers is that they can analyze vast amounts of data and identify patterns. They can be used to identify patients who are at risk of particular diseases once that patient's vitals and background are supplied, or help predict whether this patient may be subject to readmission into a hospital. However, some of these data from many sources may simply constitute what is popular at this moment as far as a treatment option, and may not be the best for the patient.

Vanderbilt University Medical Center in Nashville, Tennessee, and St. Jude's Medical Center in Memphis, Tennessee, are getting notified by computer that a particular drug may not work for a specific patient, or of a test that might help them decide on whether a patient is a candidate for a particular treatment. Medical images, radiology reports, and doctor's notes are useful for making diagnoses, but are not useful for computer programs, nor are they taken into consideration when the computer suggests a particular treatment. Ethically, it is important to have a doctor review the data or suggestions generated by a computer in order to make sure that the result is accurate. However, this may not happen all of the time, especially with the time pressure to see more patients, unless physician evaluation of a computer-generated finding becomes a rule with consequences. Who will determine what or who determined the treatment option? Thus, the line between making recommendations and making decisions becomes difficult to determine conclusively. Perhaps these computer programs should be considered as medical devices and subject to review by the U.S. Food and Drug Administration? This would be a huge and expensive task, but may become necessary in the future.

Exciting developments such as artificial limbs that respond to the brain of the patient are being developed and should help many people, especially veterans coming home from war after experiencing the loss of a limb (Figure 11.4). There is also robotic surgery or robot-assisted surgery, which allows surgeons to perform more procedures, such as rib spreading to enter the body cavity, with more flexibility, precision, strength, and control than is possible with conventional techniques.

With robotically assisted minimally invasive surgery, the surgeon does not directly move the instruments, but instead uses one of two methods to control the instrument: either a direct telemanipulator or through computer control. A telemanipulator is a remote computer-assisted instrument that allows the surgeon to perform the normal movements associated with the surgery while the robotic arm carries out the procedure. One advantage of using the computerized method is that the surgeon does not have to be present, but can be anywhere in the world, which may lead to remote surgery. Robotic surgery has been criticized for its expense, by one estimate costing $1500–$2000 more per patient. The other issue is ethical: who is then responsible for the end result if there is a problem?

The possibility that we will create artificial intelligence that rivals or exceeds human intelligence raises difficult ethical questions. It also inspires both hope and fear for the future of medicine and society.

In conclusion, numerous ethical questions remain and should be considered as personalized medicine continues to develop. International and national laws protecting all patients need to be strengthened and penalties implemented. Privacy laws need to have clear legal and financial repercussions for breaches. Issues on the applicability of personalized therapeutics for everyone should be considered and need to be addressed as personalized medicine grows. If we are to have a viable medical care system in the United States, guidelines and regulations on medical and pharmaceutical costs need to be developed by the government. It does not appear that the pharmaceutical and insurance companies alone are capable of policing themselves in order to bring down costs and guarantee full equity for patients. Some of these changes are already occurring with the Affordable Care Act and medical reimbursement based on healthy patient outcomes rather than for the number of procedures and tests performed. Patient autonomy, well-being, and equity need to be ensured. Finally, as new advances in research become available, laws/guidelines based on ethical issues for ensuring no harm comes to patients need to be anticipated, established, and maintained.

REFERENCES

Dorschner, MO, LM Amendola, EH Turner et al. 2015. Actionable exomic incidental findings in 6503 participants: Challenges of variant classification. *Genome Res* 25(3):305–15.

Fei, D. 2015. *Girl in Glass*. Bloomsbury Press USA, New York.

Guerts, AM, GJ Cost, Y Freyvert et al. 2009. Knockout rats produced using designed zinc finger nucleases. *Science* 325:433.

Hernandez, D. 2014. Artificial Intelligence is now telling doctors how to treat you. Kaiser Health *News Business* February 6, 2014.

Joly, Y, I Ngueng Feze, and J Simard. 2013. Genetic discrimination and life insurance: A systematic review of the evidence. *BMC Med* 11:25.

Kolata, G. 2015. Chinese scientists edit genes of human embryos. *New York Times*, April 24, 2015.

Lanphier, E, F Urnov, SE Haecker, M Werner, and J Smolenski. 2015. Don't edit the human germ line. *Nature* 519 (7544):410–1.

Lewis, J, W Lipworth, and I Kerridge. 2014. Ethics, evidence and economics in the pursuit of "personalized medicine." *J Pers Med* 4:137–46.

Liang, P, Y Xu, X Zhang et al. 2015. CRISPR/Cas9-mediated gene editing in human tripronuclear zygotes. *Protein Cell* 6(5):363–72.

Mackenzie, R, S Chapman, G Salkeld, and S Holding. 2008. Media influence on Herceptin subsidization in Australia: Application of the rule of rescue? *J R Soc Med* 101:305–12.

Tebas, P, D Stein, WW Tang et al. 2014. Gene editing of CCR5 in autologous CD4 T cells of persons infected with HIV. *N Engl J Med* 370(10):901–10.

Wilson, BJ and SG Nicholls. 2015. The Human Genome Project, and recent advances in personalized genomics. *Risk Manag Healthc Policy* 8:9–20.

12

Conclusions

Amazing advances have been made in science to improve medical care in the twenty-first century with the development of genomics and genetic screening, the realization of the importance of environmental factors for gene expression and inheritance through epigenetics, and the myriad new tests and pharmaceuticals that have been developed from proteomics and botanical products. On the other hand, it is premature to say that our medical system or medical institutions can deliver personalized medicine to most patients at this point in time. How can we advance personalized medicine in the future?

Let us start with what individuals can do for their own health. Let us become more involved in preventative care. If we want to achieve personalized medicine, then the patient's role in attending to their health needs to be encouraged. Part of this change needs to start in public schools where good nutrition, daily exercise, and some knowledge of human physiology and diseases need to be emphasized. We cannot relegate exercise to just afternoon programs independent of our schools, since only wealthier parents are able to afford many of these sports programs. The strength and mass of our bones are already determined by the time we leave our 20s. Therefore, exercise programs are helpful in obtaining the greatest bone mass for each individual, especially girls, who will lose more bone mass than men when they reach menopause and are more likely to develop osteoporosis. As I write this last chapter, the United States' 5–2 victory over the defending Japanese champions gave the American women's soccer team the FIFA Women's World Cup 2015 trophy. The American team's last such win was in 1999. Perhaps this achievement will inspire more young women to try out for sports, allow all young people to maintain sporting activities throughout their life, and encourage investors in women's sports. For young men, involvement in school sports, along with summer job programs, helps to keep them occupied in positive activities and also allows them to perform better in school, since a sound body leads to a sound mind.

Obesity has reached epidemic proportions in the United States, and other countries as well. Unless we teach children to make better choices in terms of food and provide nutritious and balanced meals at school, we will lose the battle against obesity and metabolic syndrome, leading to high blood pressure and diabetes. If we care about our young people and the population at large, banning unhealthy foods, such as super-sized sugary sodas as the mayor of New York City did, might be the right route to take. We have discouraged smoking cigarettes with high taxes and health warnings, and now we are faced with e-cigarettes and their high levels of nicotine and which are still addictive. The health risk of e-cigarettes needs to be addressed, along with other ways to discourage their use, especially among young people. These suggestions are just some of the changes requiring a patient's role in their own health, along with appropriate government regulations, and in order for personalized medicine to be successful and not overburden the healthcare system.

Scientific exploration, diagnosis, and treatment of the major ailments in the world—mental disorders—tragically have not been priorities. So much more work needs to be done in understanding the brain, neurobiology, and mental afflictions and on developing new therapies with fewer side effects. For example, bipolar disorder, formerly known as manic–depressive illness, is a brain and behavior disorder characterized by severe shifts in a person's mood and energy, which makes it difficult for the person to function at times. The expression of the condition is also highly varied between different individuals, and we do not know the cause of the disorder. Each year, more than 5.7 million American adults or 2.6% of the population aged 18 or older suffer from bipolar disorder. Many people live with bipolar symptoms without having it properly diagnosed and treated. This mental disorder is underdiagnosed, undertreated, and not well understood.

Cancer therapies are becoming more personalized as different subsets of particular cancers are discovered, such as luminal a, luminal b, HER-2 enriched, basal-like or triple-negative breast cancers. With the knowledge of these and other types of biomarkers on cancer cells, specific targeted approaches to cancers are being investigated and implemented. Although the most common types of cancers are treated with broadly targeted chemotherapeutic drugs that kill all fast-growing cells, it is hoped in the future that we will have better therapies that do not injure or destroy so many normal cells and cause additional medical problems for those who survive cancer. We do not know why certain individuals have so many side effects from chemotherapy for all types of cancer, while other individuals are less affected. Scientists are trying to understand this issue and to develop more targeted approaches for eradicating cancer with fewer side effects. Earlier detection of all types of cancer before it can undergo metastasis will be helpful in preventing the deleterious effects of prolonged chemotherapeutic treatments and radiation.

Personalized therapeutics must not only include devices and pharmaceuticals, but also other integrative medicine techniques for which there is some sound scientific evidence of benefit. Prolonged stress has many deleterious effects on the body, such as cardiovascular disease and overeating leading to obesity. Excessive and long-term stress leads to depression of the immune system that, in turn, can lead to more susceptibility to disease and even cancer. Exercise, mind–body therapies, meditation, and yoga are just some of the integrative therapies that have health benefits. Investment in up-and-coming research in integrative medicine should be considered for enacting personalized medical solutions to the medical issues faced by individuals. Places of work should offer stress reduction programs or facilities to improve the health and productivity of their employees. We already know that less sitting improves creativity.

Genomics, with its predictions for disease likelihood, and stem cell research for tissue engineering and regenerative medicine are exciting young fields of science and will lead to major advances in individual health outcomes. Stem cell research is in its infancy, but offers the promise of repairing and replacing injured and diseased tissues and organs. As discussed in the early chapters, the pitfall in genomics is that knowing what genes are present in an individual, as determined by sequencing DNA, does not tell us definitively if that person will develop a disease, even though one may have a mutation in a gene predisposing one to a particular disease. Environmental exposures and genetic factors, such as microRNAs, will influence the expression of that gene. At this point in time, knowledge of these factors and their repercussions is too complicated for us to make accurate predictions or to provide a mechanism for preventing the expression of a deleterious gene. How will our medical insurance companies and medical system define and pay for procedures that are for diseases that we may or may not get?

As previously mentioned, the U.S. medical system is 47th in the world in terms of timeliness of treatment, outcomes, and expense. How will personalized medicine affect this rating? Without a well-thought out plan for the development of personalized medicine, our healthcare system will not be sustainable. Without more emphasis on preventative care rather than expensive acute care, our medical system will continue to slide down in timeliness, cost, and outcomes. The Affordable Care Act has tried to improve healthcare delivery and make it more uniform so that uninsured patients receive better care than just trips to the emergency room with acute problems. Emergency rooms are very expensive and do not deal with the underlying issues of the chronic problems of cardiovascular disease, obesity, metabolic syndrome, diabetes, etc. The Affordable Care Act prevents discrimination by health insurance companies against patients with pre-existing health conditions.

Increased education on the benefits of having healthcare coverage and appropriate vaccination for preventable diseases is needed. For those with low wages, health plans need to be sustainable considering income and family needs. Given the present system, penalties for not having health insurance will rise with each subsequent year in the United States, and this is only fair when one considers that everyone ends up paying for expensive emergency room visits and paying more for medical care for the uninsured. More education on the types of medical plans and tax benefits available would help people make better decisions. This is not just an issue for the medical system, but also for our whole society. If minimum wages are increased, more families and individuals may sign up for health plans and be able to stimulate the economy through their increased purchasing power.

The medical system needs to emphasize monetary rewards for improving patients' health and increasing preventative care, rather than reimbursing physicians and hospitals for the number of procedures and tests performed. This change is already occurring in some places. We should observe other countries whose healthcare systems are more sustainable and have better ratings. Some of these countries have socialized medicine, but they may also provide programs that we may be able to incorporate into our system to improve U.S. healthcare. Our government can certainly negotiate better prices with the pharmaceutical and medical device companies for patients. Education of families on the safety and need for vaccinations is essential. Maintaining high standards in medical care and overseeing the ethical development of automated medicine is also of great concern. Automation could be helpful in decreasing medical costs, but it must always be reviewed by doctors in order to ensure ethical and appropriate treatments are administered.

Monitoring different aspects of our healthcare system, including insurance companies, private physicians, and hospitals, in order to provide fair prices, procedures, and ethical decisions will perhaps stem our steep decline in the quality of medical care. For example, the recent scandal in the Veterans Administration's (VA's) healthcare system caused our veterans in some hospitals to wait for treatment for many months. On April 30, 2014, Cable News Network (CNN) reported that at least 40 U.S. Armed Forces veterans (later confirmed at 35) died while waiting for medical care at the Phoenix, Arizona, Veterans Health Administrations facilities. The VA Office of the Inspector General is investigating, and the House of Representatives has passed legislation to fund a major criminal investigation by the Justice Department. As a result, the VA's top health official resigned under pressure. Additional VA medical centers around the nation have been identified as having similar problems and are being investigated. An internal VA audit released on June 9, 2014, found that more than 120,000 veterans were left waiting or never received care, and that schedulers were pressured to use unofficial lists or engage in inappropriate practices to make waiting times appear more favorable (Cohen 2014). Whatever the number, it is terrible that men and women who risked their lives to serve our country did not receive adequate medical treatment. Perhaps your individual medical care is excellent, but when you average out what is happening around the country and in the VA, one can understand why our medical care system is not timely, not reasonable in price, and does not have the best outcomes. It is hoped that with more oversight and penalties that include imprisonment, this will never happen again.

Increased investment in medical and scientific research in order to improve medical treatment should be a priority in our country, because we are very capable of developing creative solutions to problems in science, medicine, and bioinformatics. We have to have open minds for creative and fair solutions in order to achieve good medical care treatment for all of our citizens, even if this means sacrificing some aspects of personalized medicine and some of our personal freedoms.

An eloquent defense for more health-related research came in an op-ed article in the *New York Times*, written by former Republican Speaker of the U.S. House of Representatives, Newt Gingrich (Gingrich 2015). In his article, he justified doubling the budget of the National Institutes of Health (NIH) by suggesting that this would cut costs for healthcare, for which taxpayers currently spend $1 trillion. The NIH is an agency of the U.S. Department of Health and Human Services and is the primary agency of the government for biomedical and health-related research. It funds its own research (having about 6,000 scientists) and also an Extramural Research Program with 50,000 competitive grants and 300,000 researchers at more than 2,500 universities in basic, translational, and clinical research. It is the largest biomedical research institution in the world, and comprises 27 separate institutes and centers that conduct research in different scientific/medical areas with a total budget of $30.3 billion in 2014 (http://officeofbudget.od.nih.gov/cy.html). In fact, 145 Nobel Prize winners have received support from the NIH. The NIH's scientific accomplishments, among others, include the development of the MRI, the discovery of fluoride for preventing tooth decay, the use of lithium for bipolar disorder, and the creation of vaccines against hepatitis, *Haemophilus influenzae*, and human papillomavirus.

In the article, Newt Gingrich gives the example of the total cost of healthcare for patients with Alzheimer's disease and other dementias, for which the budget will exceed $20 trillion over the next four decades. In contrast, the NIH only has 0.8% of the cost of funds this current year dedicated to dementia research. If a small advance in medical treatment for Alzheimer's patients could delay the onset of this disease by 5 years, then we could reduce the number of Americans with Alzheimer's disease in 2050 by 42% and cut costs by a third. In fact, presently, the NIH is studying interventions in families with a genetic predisposition to early-onset Alzheimer's disease in order to prevent the disease before symptoms develop. Alzheimer's disease is only an example of the many diseases, such as diabetes, heart disease, cancer, stroke, kidney disease, and arthritis, for which we could cut medical costs and find better solutions for patient care, and even develop cures for some of these diseases.

Another goal of personalized medicine is to create or find the most appropriate types and doses of medications and/or interventions in order to deal with a person's health issue. For example, my doctors at the University of Connecticut Health Center worked very hard to build a therapeutic regimen that would rid me of cancer. July 1, 2015, was my 5-year mark since surgery, and 2016 will be 5 years from chemotherapy and radiation. Another part of my therapeutic regimen is to take an inhibitor of estrogen production (aromatase inhibitor), a daily pill, for at least 5 years in order to destroy any cancer cells with estrogen receptors. Did it work? So far, so good, but who knows the future? I am now faced with difficulties walking, which started during chemotherapy. I am in the process of determining whether this is due to degeneration of my spine or due to damage to my legs and muscles as a result of chemotherapy. Or, in my worst dreams, could I be developing a muscular/neurological disease? However, I never for one moment regretted going through chemotherapy, and I worked almost every day during those 12 weeks of treatments, although with reduced efficiency and time. During the last month of treatment, my oncologist reduced the dosage of chemotherapy, but I still could not tolerate the final weeks of treatment, so she cut out my last few treatments. As previously stated, my doctor called me a "bad responder" to the chemotherapy, since I developed so many side effects, which I still suffer from now. My doctor told me that the hope for the future is to tailor more personalized chemotherapy regimens with the hope of limiting and even preventing side effects. This personalization will require a better understanding of an individual's physiology through testing that may predict how one responds to a treatment, such as chemotherapy. Because of my personal health issues, I have become more proactive, sold my home in Connecticut, and built a house in a warmer climate. I am now eating more fish and vegetables, bicycling, walking, swimming, and practicing yoga to try and strengthen my legs, and waiting for my doctors to complete their tests to tell me what may be wrong.

REFERENCES

Cohen, T. 2014. Audit: More than 120,000 veterans waiting or never got care. *CNN*, June 10, 2014.

Gingrich, N. 2015. Double the N.I.H. budget. *New York Times*, April 22, 2015.

Glossary of scientific terms

Acetylation is when an acetyl group is transferred to different regions of amino acids, especially as polypeptides are being formed. N-acetylation occurs in 80%–90% of eukaryotic proteins, but the biological significance of this process is not completely known. Another important acetylation occurs on the lysine of histone N-termini and is a method for regulating gene transcription. Histones package the DNA of the chromatin so that it can fit into the nucleus. When the histone is acetylated, it reduces the condensation or packaging of the chromosome so that transcription can take place.

Acupuncture is a traditional Chinese technique in which a practitioner stimulates specific points on the body using thin needles inserted in the skin, and is known to alleviate certain types of pain.

Adaptive immune system or cell-mediated immune system recognizes antigens, which it processes. Once an antigen has been recognized, the adaptive immune system creates an army of immune cells designed to attack that antigen. T and B lymphocytes and macrophages are part of the army of immune cells that also lead to a memory of the encounter for future exposures to that same antigen.

Adenosine triphosphate (ATP) is an energy molecule that is produced by cellular respiration or fermentation and is used to power most cellular reactions. When powering a cellular reaction, it loses a phosphate group to become adenosine diphosphate (ADP), and then reverts back to ATP through cellular respiration or fermentation.

Adrenal glands are glands situated on top of the kidneys that secrete steroid hormones such as the androgens, the corticosteroids, and the mineralocorticoids, regulating blood pressure and electrolyte balance, and glucocorticoids, such as cortisol, regulating glycogen and lipid metabolism and immune system suppression.

Adrenal medulla is the innermost part of the adrenal gland. It secretes epinephrine (adrenaline), norepinephrine (noradrenaline), and small amounts of dopamine. It is stimulated by the sympathetic preganglionic neurons.

Adrenaline, also known as epinephrine, is a hormone and a neurotransmitter. It is secreted by the adrenal gland and is also produced by the ends of sympathetic nerve fibers.

Adrenocorticotropic hormone (ACTH) is a hormone secreted by the pituitary gland that causes increased release of cortisol, a steroid hormone that is released in response to stress or low blood sugar.

Agonist is a chemical that binds and activates a receptor to cause a biological response.

Akinesia is a loss or impairment of voluntary movement.

Aldosterone is a mineralocorticoid hormone produced by the adrenal cortex in the adrenal gland. It plays a role in the regulation of blood pressure in the kidney by increasing reabsorption of ions and water.

Algorithm is a process with a set of rules to be followed in calculations or other problem-solving operations, especially by a computer.

Allele is one of a number of alternative forms of the same gene or genetic locus, which can create different phenotypic traits. However, most alleles do not produce any visible variation.

Alpha(α)-interferon (IFN). The type I IFNs present in humans are IFN-α, IFN-β, IFN-ϵ, IFN-κ, and IFN-ω. IFNs are signaling proteins made and released by host cells in response to the presence of pathogens, such as viruses, bacteria, parasites, or tumor cells. A virus-infected cell will release interferons, causing nearby cells to increase antiviral defenses. IFN-α is also used as a drug to treat people with hepatitis C.

Alpha(α)-methyl-CoA racemase (AMACR) is an enzyme that is found to be increased in prostate cancer. About ten different variants of human AMACR have been identified from prostate cancer tissues, which arise from alternative mRNA splicing.

Alternative medicine is a medical practice that is considered to have a healing effect that is not based on evidence from scientific methodology and is used instead of traditional medicine.

Alternative splicing is when the coding regions of genes are assembled in a different way after splicing, resulting in different proteins being formed from the same gene.

Alzheimer's disease is a chronic neurodegenerative disease causing loss of memory, loss of language function, mood swings, disorientation, loss of motivation, and behavioral issues. Alzheimer's disease has an unknown cause and is characterized by loss of neurons and synapses in the brain and amyloid plaques, neurofibrillary tangles, and misfolded proteins.

Amino acids are the basic building blocks of proteins, consisting of an amine group, a carboxylic acid group, and a side chain specific to each amino acid.

Amyloids are misfolded protein fragments that form aggregates in the body. β-amyloid is a protein fragment snipped from an amyloid precursor protein (APP). In a healthy brain, these protein fragments are broken down and eliminated.

Androgens are natural or synthetic compounds that bind to androgen receptors that control the development and maintenance of male sex characteristics. The most commonly known androgen is testosterone.

Angiogenesis is a physiological process by which new blood vessels form from pre-existing vessels.

Antagonists are receptor ligands or drugs that will bind to a receptor without causing a biological response and will block the action of an agonist.

Anterior cingulated cortex is the frontal portion of the brain that controls autonomic functions like blood pressure and heart rate, and also cognitive functions such as decision making, empathy, impulse control, and emotion.

Antibodies are proteins that are produced by the immune system to bind foreign antigens and pathogens and mark them for elimination.

Antidiuretic hormone (ADH) or vasopressin is a hormone that helps to retain water in the body by increasing water reabsorption in the kidneys and also constricts blood vessels.

Antigen is any substance (for example, foreign substances from the environment, such as chemicals, bacteria, viruses, or pollen; an antigen may also be formed inside the body, as with bacterial toxins or tissue cells) that causes the immune system to produce antibodies against it.

Antioxidant is a molecule that inhibits oxidation reactions, which are reactions that involve the loss of electrons. Oxidation can produce free radicals that can start reactions within cells, leading to cell damage.

Apoptosis is the process of programmed cell death.

Argonaute proteins are a family of proteins that are involved in RNA silencing and are a component of the RNA-induced silencing complex (RISC) in epigenetics.

Aromatase is an enzyme responsible for the biosynthesis of estrogens.

Aromatherapy is an adjuvant therapy in integrative medicine that uses the scent of plant materials and oils to alter a person's mood and psychological or physical well-being.

Arteries are blood vessels that carry the blood away from the heart. Most arteries carry oxygenated blood, but there are two exceptions: the pulmonary and the umbilical arteries.

Arteriosclerosis is the hardening of the medium and large arteries frequently from fatty plaques and cholesterol and can cause severe health risks, including heart attack.

Assay is a biochemical or medical method for measuring the functioning of an analyte (measured target).

Atherosclerosis is a form of arteriosclerosis (hardening of the arteries) that is caused by white blood cells accumulating in the artery wall due to chronic inflammation. Low-density lipoproteins (LDLs) typically bring triglycerides and cholesterol to the artery wall without high-density lipoproteins (HDLs) removing them.

ATPases are enzymes that catalyze the breakdown of ATP to ADP plus phosphate and use the resulting energy to catalyze other reactions.

Attention deficit disorder (ADD) and attention deficit-hyperactivity disorder (ADHD) are disorders characterized by inattention, hyperactivity, and impulsive behavior. These symptoms can affect learning, behavior, and emotional responses. Although mostly diagnosed in children, ADD can carry over into adulthood.

Autism is a developmental disease that causes impaired social interaction and verbal and non-verbal communication and repetitive behavior.

Autogenic training is a relaxation technique that involves short daily practice sessions, in which a practitioner repeats a set of visualizations that induce relaxation in a person.

Autoimmunity is an immune response in which an organism activates its immune system against its own cells and tissues.

Autonomic nervous system (ANS) is the part of the peripheral nervous system that regulates the function of the internal organs.

B

B lymphocytes or B cells are immune cells that are primarily responsible for the production of antibodies when exposed to an antigen. They present antigens to other cells and retain humoral "immunity" to diseases by forming memory B cells. B lymphocytes also release cytokines.

Basal layer is the deepest of the five layers of skin cells and is primarily made up of basal keratinocyte cells (skin cells), which are effectively the stem cells of the skin.

Basal side of a cell is the region of the plasma membrane that faces the underlying connective tissue.

Base. In DNA, there are four different bases: adenine (A) and guanine (G) are purines, and cytosine (C) and thymine (T) are the smaller pyrimidines. RNA also contains four bases. Three of these are the same as in DNA: A, G, and C. Uracil (U) is the fourth base found in RNA. The base pairs are AT or CG.

β-cells are cells in the pancreas that are responsible for the production of insulin, which regulates sugar levels. In type 1 diabetes, the β-cells are attacked by the immune system.

Biofeedback is a technique that trains a person to improve their health by controlling particular bodily processes that normally happen involuntarily, such as heart rate, blood pressure, muscle tension, and skin temperature.

Bioinformatics is a field that develops methods and software for understanding biological data. It is a combination of computer science, statistics, mathematics, and engineering.

Biomarkers are measurable substances or characteristics in the human body that can be used to monitor the presence of a chemical in the body or biological responses.

Biomaterials are objects, such as metals, that interact with a biological system and most often are used to repair defects in the tissue.

Biopsy is a sampling of cells from a tissue used to determine the presence or extent of a disease.

Biostatistics is the use of statistics to quantify biological processes.

Bipolar disease is a common disorder that is characterized by mood swings ranging from depressive lows to manic highs. There are more than 3 million cases in the United States per year.

Blastocysts are formations of cells in the early development of an animal. Embryonic stem cells are taken from this phase of development.

Blood pressure is the pressure exerted by the blood on the walls of the blood vessels. It is composed of the systolic or contractile pressure and the diastolic or resting pressure.

Body mass index (BMI) is a mathematical formula that is based on a person's height and weight, and is used to measure fatness.

Bone marrow is the spongy tissue, called hematopoietic tissue, inside the bones that produces red blood cells, platelets, and most white blood cells in mammals. It also contains fat cells and numerous blood vessels.

Bone mineral density (BMD) is the amount of bone mineral per square centimeter of bone.

Bone morphogenetic proteins (BMPs) are a family of growth factors that are important in determining tissue architecture throughout the body, but are particularly studied in bone and cartilage. Recombinant human BMPs, especially BMP-2, are used in orthopedic applications, such as spinal fusions, non-unions, and oral surgery.

Bradykinesia is slowness of movement frequently associated with Parkinson's disease. It is not slowness in initiation of movement, only in the actual execution of the movement.

Brainstem is the posterior part of the brain where the brain connects to the spinal cord. It is responsible for the regulation of many autonomic functions and maintaining consciousness.

Buddhism is a nontheistic philosophy or way of life that encompasses a variety of traditions, beliefs, and spiritual practices, largely based on teachings attributed to Gautama Buddha. According to Buddhist tradition, the Buddha lived and taught in the northeastern part of India sometime between the sixth and fourth centuries BCE. He developed the philosophy of Buddhism.

C

C-reactive protein is a protein that is made by the liver and is found in blood. C-reactive protein levels increase in response to inflammation in order to activate the complement (immune) system.

Caffeine is a methylxanthine protein found in coffee, soft drinks, and some seeds, nuts, or beans. It is a central nervous system stimulant and a psychoactive drug.

Calcinosis is the creation of calcium deposits in any tissue. It can occur from soft tissue damage (dystrophic), a calcium imbalance (metastatic), or through an unknown cause, accumulating near the joints (tumoral).

Calorie is approximately the amount of energy that is needed to increase the temperature of 1 g of water by 1°C at a pressure of 1 atmosphere.

Capillaries are the smallest blood vessels in the body that transmit most of the nutrients between the blood and surrounding tissues.

Carbohydrates are biological molecules consisting of one carbon, hydrogen, and oxygen that usually have two hydrogens for each oxygen. In biochemistry, a carbohydrate often refers to a saccharide, which includes sugars, starches, and cellulose.

Carcinoma is a cancer of epithelial cells.

Castration is any process, either surgical, chemical, or otherwise, by which a biological male loses use of his testicles.

Catecholamine is a molecule that has a catechol (benzene ring with two hydroxyl groups), including epinephrine, norepinephrine, and dopamine. It is produced by the adrenal medulla and sympathetic nervous system.

Caudate–putamen are two structures in the brain made up of the caudate nucleus and the putamen. The caudate–putamen regulates learning and movement and is linked with degenerative neural disorders such as Parkinson's disease.

Cell sorting is a method of separating cells according to their phenotypic properties.

Census Bureau is the organization that produces statistics about the American people and economy.

Central nervous system consists of the brain and spinal cord.

Cerebral cortex is the outside of the cerebrum in the brain and is responsible for memory, attention, perception, awareness, thought, language, and consciousness.

Cerebral ischemia is a condition in which there is lack of blood flow to the brain and can cause death of brain tissue, such as in a stroke.

Chemiluminescence is the production of light from a chemical reaction.

Chemokines are cell signaling molecules or cytokines that are secreted by cells to induce chemotaxis in neighboring cells. Chemotaxis is a process by which cells move according to the presence of a chemical (i.e., chemokine) in their surrounding environment.

Chemotherapy is a cancer treatment that uses anticancer drugs to eliminate the malignant cells or to treat symptoms.

Cholecalciferol, or vitamin D_3, is synthesized by the body and is a precursor to calcitriol, which regulates many enzymes in the body by binding to the vitamin D receptor in almost every cell.

Cholecystokinin receptors are G-protein-coupled receptors that bind to cholecystokinin, which promotes the pathways responsible for the digestion of fat and is also linked to the tolerance of and withdrawal from opiate drugs.

Cholesterol is a lipid molecule that is required in the synthesis of cell membranes and is a major cause of heart disease when there are elevated levels in the blood.

Chromosomes are wound up structures of DNA bound by histones and linked in the center by a centromere. They carry the genes of an organism.

Chronic lymphocytic leukemia is the most common type of leukemia, a cancer of the white blood cells, in particular the B lymphocytes.

Circulatory system is an organ system that transports blood in order to deliver nutrients and removes harmful waste from the cells in the body.

Cirrhosis is the scarring of liver tissue that results in a malfunctioning liver.

Clustered regularly interspaced short palindromic repeats (CRISPR) is a bacteria-derived system that uses RNA in order to recognize specific human DNA sequences and then uses an endonuclease, Cas9, to cut the required sequence for genetic manipulation. The whole complex is called CRISPR/Cas9. Cas9 is an abbreviation for CRISPR-associated protein 9.

Codons are sequences of three DNA or RNA nucleotides that correspond to specific amino acids or stop signals during protein synthesis.

Cognitive–behavioral therapy is a type of psychotherapy that focuses on correcting maladaptive thoughts and actions in order to relieve symptoms of mental illness.

Complement system is part of the innate immune system that helps to kill pathogens by activation of the membrane attack complex (MAC) in response to antibody–antigen complexes, a consistent background activation, or the lectin pathway. It helps antibodies and phagocytic cells to clear pathogens from an organism.

Complementary medicine is a type of medicine that involves healing practices and products that work in conjunction with traditional medicine.

Connective tissue is a tissue in our bodies that supports, connects, or separates different types of tissues and organs. Connective tissue is found everywhere in the body except the central nervous system.

Copy number variants are forms of structural variation in the DNA that result in the cell having an abnormal number of copies of one or more regions of the DNA.

Corticosteroids are chemicals that are produced in the adrenal cortex that mediate many biological processes such as stress responses, immune responses, inflammation, carbohydrate and protein metabolism, electrolyte levels, and behavior.

Corticotropin-releasing factor (CRF) is produced by the hypothalamus and is a neurotransmitter involved in stress responses.

Cortisol is a glucocorticoid hormone that is produced in the adrenal cortex in response to stress or low blood glucose. Cortisol suppresses the immune system, modulates bone formation, and increases carbohydrate, protein, and fat metabolism in order to increase blood glucose.

Cyclins are a family of proteins that control the progression of cells through the cell cycle for cell division by activating cyclin-dependent kinase (Cdk) enzymes.

Cystic fibrosis is a genetic disorder that results in thick mucus, leading to an inability to breathe, increased infections, growth interference, fatty stool, clubbing of the digits, and many other symptoms.

Cystic fibrosis transmembrane conductance regulator (CFTR) is a membrane protein that transfers chloride ions. People who are homozygous for the mutation to the CFTR gene exhibit cystic fibrosis.

Cytokines are chemicals that are part of cell signaling pathways and include chemokines, interferons, interleukins, lymphokines, and tumor necrosis factor, but not hormones or growth factors.

Cytoskeleton is a matrix inside the cell that gives the cell its structure and helps to organize many cellular functions inside the cell. There are three main proteins that the cytoskeleton consists of: microfilaments, microtubules, and intermediate filaments. Part of the cytoskeleton is contractile, while other components are involved in the movement of molecules within the cell and cell signaling.

D

Demethylation is a chemical process that results in the removal of a methyl group ($-CH_3$) from a molecule.

Dendritic cells are antigen-presenting cells of the immune system. Their main function is to process antigen material and present it to T cells. They act as messengers between the innate and the adaptive immune systems.

Deoxyribonucleic acid (DNA) is the genetic code responsible for containing the heritable information of an organism and instructions for producing proteins.

Deoxyribose is a simple sugar, consisting of a ribose that has lost an oxygen atom.

Depolarization is the process by which cells, which are usually electronegative internally, rapidly become electropositive for a very short period of time. This process is part of cellular signaling between neurons.

Diabetes mellitus, commonly referred to as diabetes, is a group of metabolic diseases in which there is high blood sugar over a prolonged period of time.

Diabetes type 1 results from an autoimmune reaction of the body to the β-cells in the pancreas, which produce insulin, and the disease manifests mostly in juveniles.

Diabetes type 2 results from growing insensitivity to insulin, which is mediated by poor diet and genetics. Diabetes type 2 mostly manifests in adulthood.

Diagnostic and Statistical Manual of Mental Disorders (DSM) is a book that gives the criteria for diagnosing mental disorders and is published by the American Psychiatric Association.

Diploid describes a cell that has two homologous copies of each chromosome. Diploidy in mammals describes the condition of healthy somatic cells.

DNA fingerprinting or DNA profiling is a test for certain genetic markers that can identify specific individuals.

DNA polymerases are enzymes that create DNA by assembling nucleotides, the building blocks of DNA. DNA polymerases are essential to DNA replication and usually work in pairs to create two identical DNA strands from a single original DNA molecule.

Dominance is a genetic relationship between alleles in which the dominant allele determines the phenotype of an organism.

Dopamine is a neurotransmitter that performs many roles within the brain, including reward-motivated behavior. Other brain dopamine systems are involved in motor control and in controlling the release of several other important hormones.

Dopaminergic neurons are neurons that are activated by dopamine.

Dual x-ray absorptiometry (DXA) is a technique that measures bone mineral density by using two x-rays of differing frequencies: one x-ray measures total bone mass, and then the soft tissue mass from the other scan is subtracted out of the total.

E

Ectoderm is a germ layer in the early embryo that resides on the outside of the embryo. It gives rise to the nervous system, parts of the skull, and the epidermis.

Elastic fibers are bundles of proteins that are able to stretch, and are found in connective tissue and arteries.

Endocrine system consists of the glands that secrete hormones into the blood and regulate metabolism, growth and development, tissue function, sexual function, reproduction, sleep, and mood, etc.

Endoderm is a germ layer on the inside of the early embryo. It gives rise to the respiratory tract, the gastrointestinal tract, the endocrine system, the auditory system, and the urinary system.

Endonucleases are enzymes that cleave the phosphodiester bond within a polynucleotide chain. Some cut DNA in nonspecific regions, while many, typically called restriction endonucleases or restriction enzymes, cleave only at very specific nucleotide sequences.

Endorphins are opioid neuropeptides that are naturally produced in the body. Opiate drugs mimic their effect.

Endotoxemia is the presence of lipopolysaccharides in the blood that produce inflammation. Lipopolysaccharides are found on the outside of bacteria and elicit immune responses.

Energy medicine is a type of integrative medicine in which practitioners use the human biofield to promote health and well-being in a patient. The exact composition of the human biofield is not known.

Enteric nervous system is the part of the nervous system that regulates the gastrointestinal tract.

Enzymes are biological catalysts. They help to speed up chemical reactions in the body.

Epidermal growth factor is a protein that promotes cell growth, survival, and differentiation.

Epigenetics is a scientific field in which the variability in an organism's phenotype (active traits) is found not to be due to genetics, but rather due to modifications to protein production and gene expression by modifying the DNA without changing the base coding.

Epinephrine (see **adrenaline**).

Epithelium is a type of tissue that lines the surfaces of the body and is involved in protection, secretion, and absorption.

Estrogen is a hormone that is the primary female sex hormone and helps control the reproductive cycle and female reproductive organs. It also has a role in metabolism, fat storage, the maintenance of blood vessels and skin, bone formation and resorption, coagulation, lung function, and lipid synthesis, and it affects the gastrointestinal tract.

Ethics in science involves the application of fundamental ethical principles to scientific research. These include the design and implementation of research involving human, animal, and cell experimentation.

Exons are nucleotide sequences within a gene that are joined together into the final mature RNA after splicing out the exon. RNA splicing takes place as part of the RNA processing pathway that follows transcription and precedes translation.

Exosomes are cell-derived vesicles that are present in biological fluids, including blood, urine, and the cultured media of cell cultures.

F

Familial dysautonomia is a genetic disorder that affects the development and survival of particular nerve cells.

Fatty acids are hydrophobic molecules that are the basic building blocks of a fat. They are either saturated (carbon atoms linked together with single bonds) or unsaturated (carbon atoms linked by double or triple bonds) and are important sources of fuel for the body.

Fiber is a type of carbohydrate that the body cannot digest. Most carbohydrates are broken down into sugar molecules, but fiber passes through the body undigested and helps regulate the use of sugars by preventing hunger and higher blood sugar. Sources of fiber are whole fruits, vegetables, whole grains, and beans.

Fibrillin-1 is an elastic connective tissue protein. Mutations in this protein are associated with Marfan syndrome and a few other genetic diseases.

Fibrosis is the thickening and scarring of connective tissue, usually as a result of injury.

Fluorophores or fluorochromes are fluorescent chemical compounds that can emit and re-emit light upon light excitation.

Food and Drug Administration (FDA) or USFDA is a federal agency of the U.S. Department of Health and Human Services. The FDA is responsible for protecting and promoting public health through the regulation and supervision of food safety, tobacco products, dietary supplements, prescription and over-the-counter pharmaceutical drugs, vaccines, blood transfusions, medical devices, electromagnetic radiation-emitting devices, cosmetics, animal foods and feed, and veterinary products.

Forensic science is the application of science in law enforcement. Scientific evidence is collected, analyzed, and preserved to solve a particular crime.

G

Gametes are cells that contain half of the DNA of an organism and bind with another organism's gamete during sexual reproduction.

γ-aminobutyric acid (GABA) is the main neurotransmitter responsible for reducing neuronal excitability.

Gangrene is a condition caused by a lack of blood supply to an area of the body, causing the death of cells in the affected area.

Gas chromatography is a scientific technique used to separate and analyze chemicals using a gas in order to move the chemicals apart.

Genes are lengths of DNA that are responsible for the production of a given protein.

Genetics is the study of genes and heredity.

Genome is the set of genes in a particular organism.

Genome-wide association study (GWAS) are whole-genome studies of organisms that determine whether or not a particular mutation is involved with a specific trait.

Genomics is the part of genetics that uses recombinant DNA, sequencing, and bioinformatics in order to analyze the complete genome.

Gleason grading system is a histology scale that defines the prognosis of men with prostate cancer.

Glucocorticoids are a class of steroid hormones that are responsible for reducing inflammation and are found in almost every vertebrate cell. They also have a role in glucose metabolism and are synthesized in the adrenal cortex.

Gluconeogenesis is a metabolic pathway that makes glucose from non-carbohydrate substrates.

Glucocorticoid responsive element (GRE) is a particular DNA sequence found in many genes that can activate or inhibit gene transcription when glucocorticoids bind to their receptors.

Glucose is a sugar with the molecular formula $C_6H_{12}O_6$. Glucose is a very important source of energy for cellular respiration. Glucose is stored in cells as glycogen.

Glutamate is an amino acid that is also known as glutamic acid and plays a very important role in neural activation.

Granulocytes are a type of white blood cell (neutrophils, eosinophils, and basophils) that help the body fight bacterial infections.

Growth hormone, or somatotropin, is a hormone that stimulates growth, cell reproduction, and regeneration.

Guided imagery is an integrative medicine technique that uses words and music in order to evoke positive imaginary scenarios in a person and so bring about a beneficial effect.

H

Helix is a curve in three-dimensional space. The double helix in the DNA molecule consists of two intertwined helices.

Hemangioma is a benign tumor of the endothelial cells in blood vessels.

Hematocrit is the volume of red blood cells in blood. Low hematocrit is associated with anemia and high hematocrit is known as polycythemia.

Heme is a cofactor consisting of an iron Fe^{2+} (ferrous) ion contained in the center of a large heterocyclic organic ring called a porphyrin. Hemes are most commonly recognized as components of hemoglobin, the red pigment in blood, but are also found in a number of other biologically important hemoproteins.

Hepatitis C is a viral disease of the liver that can lead to cirrhosis (scarring of the liver) or liver cancer.

HER-2 receptor is a cellular receptor that is similar to human epidermal growth factor, which is a marker of the more aggressive types of breast cancer.

Heterochromatin is a tightly packed form of DNA that plays a role in gene expression.

High-density lipoproteins (HDLs) are chemicals that consist of amino acids and fatty acids that circulate in the blood and are responsible for removing harmful low-density lipoproteins (LDLs) from the bloodstream.

Hinduism is the dominant religion or way of life in South Asia, particularly India. Although Hinduism contains different philosophies, it is united by shared concepts, texts, rituals, cosmology, and pilgrimage to sacred sites.

Hippocampus is a portion of the brain that is responsible for short- and long-term memory.

Histones are proteins that are major components of chromatin that wrap up DNA, making it more difficult to transcribe or rendering it inactive.

Holistic medicine is a medical practice in which all aspects of a person's needs, including psychological, physical, and social needs, are considered in disease and health.

Homeostasis is a state in which the body remains relatively stable.

Hormones are any members of a class of signaling molecules produced by glands and are transported by the circulatory system to distant target organs in order to regulate physiology and behavior.

Human biofield therapies or energy medicine is a type of integrative medicine technique in which practitioners use the human biofield to promote health and well-being in a patient. The exact composition of the human biofield is not known, but it is thought to include electromagnetic energy from the body.

Hybrid mice are produced by mating mice from two different inbred strains.

Hydrogenated vegetable oil is an oil extracted from vegetables that has hydrogen atoms added to the oil, thereby turning unsaturated fats into trans-saturated fats, which differ from the naturally occurring cis-saturated fats. "Trans fats" are associated with heart disease.

Hydrotherapy is a type of integrative medicine technique that involves the use of water for relaxation, pain relief, and treatment.

Hydroxyl radical, ·HO, is the neutral form of the hydrogen ion (HO^-). Hydroxyl radicals are highly reactive and consequently short-lived.

Hypercalcemia is the presence of excess calcium ions in the blood that can be indicative of other diseases.

Hypothalamus is a portion of the brain that releases hormones in order to link the nervous system to the endocrine system via the pituitary gland. The hypothalamus controls body temperature, hunger, behaviors such as parenting and attachment behaviors, thirst, fatigue, sleep, and circadian rhythms.

I

Immune system is the group of cells and organs involved with protecting an organism from disease.

Immunoglobulin G (IgG) is a type of antibody with two antigen binding sites. IgG represents approximately 75% of the serum antibodies in humans and is the most common antibody in the circulation. IgG is produced and released by plasma B cells.

Immunohistochemistry is a technique that detects antigens of interest in tissue sections by using antibodies against the antigen and then using various methods to detect the antigen–antibody complex through different means, including fluorescence, visible light, or radioactivity, which can be quantified.

Impotence is a condition in which a male is unable to maintain or establish an erection.

In utero is a Latin phrase that means "in the uterus."

In vitro is a Latin phrase that is used in science to describe studies that are performed with cells or biological molecules outside of their normal situation; for example, cells in artificial culture media or proteins in a solution.

Incontinency is the partial or total loss of the ability to control urination and/or defecation.

Innate immune system is a part of the immune system that comprises the cells and mechanisms that defend the body from infection by other organisms.

Institutional Review Boards (IRBs) are committees that determine whether or not an experiment is ethical based on the possible benefits to science versus the detrimental effects on the studied organisms.

Insular cortex is a portion of the brain involved with consciousness, emotion, and homeostasis.

Insulin is a hormone that regulates the metabolism of carbohydrates and fats and controls the glucose levels in the blood.

Integrative medicine. The Academic Consortium for Integrative Medicine and Health defines integrative medicine as: "Integrative medicine and health reaffirms the importance of the relationship between practitioner and patient, focuses on the whole person, is informed by evidence, and makes use of all appropriate therapeutic and lifestyle approaches, healthcare and disciplines to achieve optimal health and healing."

Interferons are a group of signaling proteins that respond to pathogens. α-interferon is used as a treatment for hepatitis C.

Interleukin-1 is a cytokine that belongs to a family of 11 cytokines that are produced by specific cells in the regulation of immune and inflammatory responses to infections or sterile wounds.

International unit (IU) is a universal measurement of biological substances. This number varies based on the specific substance being measured.

Intrauterine growth restriction is a condition in which an unborn baby is smaller than it should be because it is not growing at a normal rate inside the womb.

Introns are nucleotide sequences within a gene that are removed by RNA splicing during the formation of the final RNA product in transcription. Sequences that are joined together in the final mature RNA after RNA splicing are exons. RNA splicing takes place as part of the RNA processing pathway that follows transcription and precedes translation.

Ions are atoms or molecules in which the total number of electrons does not equal the total number of protons, giving the atom or molecule a net positive or negative electrical charge.

Iron is a mineral that is important for our body. For example, iron is part of hemoglobin, which carries oxygen from our lungs throughout our bodies. Iron helps our muscles store and use oxygen. Iron is also part of many other proteins and enzymes.

Irritable bowel syndrome (IBS) is a disease of the colon with indeterminate cause, which produces diarrhea, constipation, bloating, and/or abdominal pain.

J

Jainism is an ancient Indian philosophy that prescribes a path of non-injury towards all living beings. Practitioners believe non-injury and self-control are means of liberation from the cycle of birth and death.

K

Kilocalorie (kcal) is the energy required to raise 1000 g of water by 1°C. A dietary calorie is actually a kilocalorie.

Kinetin is a type of cytokinin, a class of plant hormone that promotes cell division. It was also found to have therapeutic potential for stem cells from patients with familial dysautonomia.

Knockout mice are mice that have had a gene or genes inactivated or removed.

L

Laser capture microdissection is a scientific technique that uses a laser coupled to a microscope in order to focus on a tissue on a slide so as to isolate and study particular groups of cells or single cells. The cells of interest are "cut out" from the adjacent tissue and they are extracted utilizing noncontact microdissection.

Law of independent assortment is a rule in genetics that states that each allele is inherited separately from any other allele when two organisms are crossed. This is not true in all situations: some alleles are linked and are frequently inherited together.

Law of segregation is a rule in genetics that states that each individual has a set of two alleles for each trait, which are separated during meiosis and recombined during fertilization to form a new organism.

Lectins are carbohydrate-binding proteins that are highly specific for sugar moieties. Lectins recognize particular sugar-containing moieties on cells. Lectins also mediate the attachment and binding of bacteria and viruses to their intended targets.

Leukemia is a cancer of the bone marrow that results in high numbers of abnormal white blood cells.

Liaison Committee on Medical Education (LCME) is an accrediting body for educational programs at schools of medicine in the United States and Canada.

Ligament is a connective tissue that connects bones together.

Limbic system of the brain is a set of brain structures associated with emotion, behavior, motivation, long-term memory, and the sense of smell.

Lipids are polymers of fatty acids. They can be fats, waxes, sterols and fat-soluble vitamins, mono-, di-, or triglycerides, phospholipids, etc. Their function is to store energy, and they are involved in cell signaling and have structural functions, such as in cell membranes.

Lipoproteins are biochemical assemblies or particles that contain both proteins and lipids.

Long-QT syndrome is an inherited or acquired condition in which the heart is in a relaxed state for too long after a heartbeat during the QT phase. This can lead to fainting, heart attacks, and death.

Low-density lipoproteins (LDLs) are chemicals composed of amino acids and fatty acids that circulate in the blood. Their build up in the circulatory system is associated with heart attacks and stroke.

Lumen is the internal part of a tube, such as an intestine or artery.

Luteinizing hormone (LH) is a hormone produced in the gonadotrophic cells in the pituitary gland that stimulate ovulation. (Gonadotropes are endocrine cells in the anterior pituitary that produce the gonadotropins, such as follicle-stimulating hormone and LH.)

Luteinizing hormone-releasing hormone (LHRH), or gonadotropin-releasing hormone (GnRH), is a neurohormone consisting of ten amino acids that is produced in the hypothalamus. LHRH stimulates the synthesis and secretion of the two hormones—luteinizing hormone and follicle-stimulating hormone—by the anterior pituitary gland.

Lymph is the fluid that circulates in the lymphatic system that is important in immune responses and protein regulation.

Lymph nodes are organs of the lymphatic system that are distributed throughout the body and are integral parts of the immune response.

Lymphocytes are white blood cells of the immune system consisting of natural killer (NK) cells, T cells, and B cells.

Lymphoma is a type of cancer of lymphatic cells.

M

Macrophages are a type of white blood cell in the immune system that engulf cellular debris, foreign substances, microbes, etc., in a process called phagocytosis. They are found in essentially all tissues.

Macular degeneration is a medical condition that results in a loss of vision in the center of the eye because of retinal damage.

Magnetic resonance imaging (MRI) is a diagnostic tool that uses magnetic fields, radio waves, and a computer to image the body.

Mammograms are diagnostic tests using low-energy x-rays in order to examine the human breast. The goal of mammography is the early detection of breast cancer, typically through the detection of characteristic masses and/or microcalcifications.

Mantras are repeated phrases, either expressed audibly or inaudibly, which help with meditation.

Marfan disease is a genetic disorder of the connective tissue that results in abnormally tall individuals who frequently have defects of the heart valve, aorta, lungs, eyes, dural sac around the spinal cord, skeleton, and soft palate.

Mass spectroscopy is a technique that identifies the amount and type of chemicals in a sample using the mass of the given chemicals.

Mastectomy is the removal of the breast, which is frequently used as a treatment for breast cancer.

Meditation is part of integrative medicine and it is the practice by which an individual trains the mind or induces a state of consciousness that quiets the mind by acknowledging the present state without including past or future events. Meditation refers to a broad variety of practices that include techniques designed to promote relaxation, build internal energy or life force, and develop compassion, love, patience, generosity, and forgiveness.

Meiosis is the process of cell division in the ovaries or testicles resulting in a monoploid germ cell.

Melanoma is a skin cancer of the melanocytes or pigment cells of the skin.

Menopause is a process that is defined as occurring 12 months after a woman's last menstrual period and marks the end of menstrual cycles. Menopause can happen in a woman's 40s or 50s, but the average age is 51 in the United States. Menopause is a natural biological process.

Meridians are involved in traditional Chinese medicine dealing with a network of paths in the body through which the life energy known as "qi" flows.

Mesoderm is a part of a developing embryo located in the middle of the embryo. It gives rise to muscle cells and many other cell types.

Messenger RNA (mRNA) is a ribonucleic acid that is transcribed from the DNA and usually codes for proteins.

Meta-analysis is the statistical method of combining the statistics from multiple studies.

Metabolic syndrome is a disease of energy utilization and storage that consists of three out of the following five conditions: obesity, high blood pressure, elevated fasting glucose, high triglycerides, and low high-density lipoproteins.

Metabolites are small molecules that participate in chemical processes in the body.

Metabolome is the complete set of small-molecule chemicals found in a given biological system.

Metabolomics is the scientific study of the chemical processes involving metabolites, such as the unique chemical fingerprints that specific cellular processes create.

Metastasis is the spread of cancer from one part of the body to another.

Methylation of DNA is the chemical alteration of DNA that results in the inactivation of a specific gene. A methyl group is added to a substrate or the substitution of an atom or group with a methyl group occurs.

Microarrays are synthesized, two-dimensional maps or "chips" designed to detect given DNA sequences in a sample. Microarrays for specific proteins and other factors are also available.

Microbes are microscopic single-celled or multicellular organisms.

Microgram is one billionth of a gram.

MicroRNA (miRNA) is a small non-coding RNA that silences other RNAs.

Mindfulness is a state of mind in which a person pays attention only to the present moment with a non-judging attitude of acceptance.

Mineralocorticoids are a class of steroid hormones that are responsible for mineral and water level regulation. The primary mineralocorticoid is aldosterone.

Minerals are naturally occurring substances that are solid and inorganic (see Table 4.3 in Chapter 4). The body uses minerals for many different jobs, including building bones, making hormones, and regulating the heartbeat.

Mitosis is the separation of one cell to produce two with the exception of germ cells.

Mole is a unit of measurement for the amount of a substance. It is defined as the amount of any chemical substance that contains as many atoms, molecules, ions, or electrons as there are atoms in 12 g of pure carbon-12. This number is expressed by the Avogadro constant, which has a value of $6.02214129 \times 10^{23}$.

Molecular biology is a branch of biology that deals with the molecular basis of biological activity.

Monocytes are white blood cells that play many roles in immune function, including moving to sites of inflammation and replication to form macrophages.

Morbidity is the existence of a certain disease state in an individual.

Mortality is the death of an organism.

Mutations are changes in the DNA of a given organism.

Myocardial infarction, also known as a heart attack, is the stopping of blood flow to the heart.

Myocytes are long muscle cells.

Myoepithelial cells are cells that are usually found in glands and have the ability to contract and expel secretions.

N

Nanoparticles are particles that are between 1 and 100 nm in diameter.

National Institutes of Health (NIH) is a biomedical research facility that is a part of the U.S. Department of Health and Human Services. It conducts its own research and also funds about 30% of the research in the United States.

Natural killer cells are cytotoxic lymphocytes of the immune system that play a major role in the host-rejection of both tumors and virally infected cells.

Neurofibrillary tangles are markers of Alzheimer's disease that consist of hyperphosphorylated tau proteins.

Neurons are cells that conduct signals throughout the nervous system.

Neuropeptides are small proteins that are used in the nervous system in order to modulate nerve activity.

Neurotransmitters are chemicals produced by neurons to communicate with other neurons across the synapse between them, or with other cells, such as muscle or gland cells.

Nevus is a medical term used to describe moles or chronic lesions of the skin or mucosa. These lesions are commonly named birthmarks or beauty marks. Nevi are benign by definition. However, 25% of malignant melanomas (skin cancers) arise from pre-existing nevi. A capillary nevus is a vascular anomaly that occurs in about 10% of all births. Some can be very extensive.

Nocebos are therapies or substances that produce a negative effect on a patient despite being inert. The opposite of a nocebo is a placebo.

Noncoding DNA or RNA is DNA or RNA that does not code for proteins.

Norepinephrine (adrenaline) is a neurotransmitter and hormone that is released from the sympathetic nervous system and affects the heart and brain.

Nuclear magnetic resonance (NMR) imaging is a form of imaging technique using electromagnetic radiation that picks up electromagnetic emissions from cell nuclei in order to form an image. The application of NMR is best known to the general public as magnetic resonance imaging for medical diagnosis and magnetic resonance microscopy in research settings.

Nuclear transfer is part of cloning. It involves the removal of the nucleus from an egg and then replacing it with the nucleus of an older donor cell that scientists want cloned, which occurs when that egg divides.

Nucleotides are the building blocks of DNA and RNA.

Nucleus is the organelle in animal cells that contains the DNA and proteins associated with transcription and regulation of transcription.

Nucleus accumbens is a part of the brain that is involved in motivation, pleasure, and reward.

Nutrition is a scientific field that interprets the interaction of nutrients and other substances in food in relation to the growth, reproduction, health, and disease of an organism.

O

Obesity is a condition in which there is too much body fat and it is detrimental to health. A body mass index (BMI; obtained by dividing a person's weight by the square of their height) above 30 indicates obesity. A BMI measurement of 25–30 is considered overweight.

Oncogenes are genes that have the potential to cause cancer.

Oocytes are the female germ cells, more commonly known as eggs.

Opiates belong to a large biosynthetic family of benzylisoquinoline alkaloids. They are named opiates because they are similar to naturally occurring alkaloids found in the opium poppy. The major psychoactive opiates are morphine, codeine, and thebaine.

Opioids are chemicals, such as morphine, which have similar effects as opiates on the body, such as pain relief, intoxication, and respiratory depression.

Orbitofrontal cortex is a part of the prefrontal cortex of the brain that is involved in decision making and other brain functions, such as sensory integration.

Osmoregulation is the regulation of the osmotic pressure, which is the pressure between two different water gradients that are trying to equalize. Osmoregulation plays an important part in hydration of cells and tissues.

Osteoarthritis is a joint disease resulting from the breakdown of cartilage that results in pain and stiffness.

Osteoporosis is a disease resulting from low bone mass that increases the risk of bone fracture.

Osteosarcoma is a cancer of the bone.

Oxytocin is a hormone that is produced by the hypothalamus and is considered to be a neuromodulator in sexual reproduction, childbirth, and social recognition and bonding.

P

Pancreas is an organ in the endocrine system that produces hormones, including insulin. The hormones and enzymes secreted by the pancreas help in digestion of carbohydrates, lipids and proteins, and control blood glucose levels.

Parasympathetic nervous system is the part of the nervous system that is responsible for regulating resting, non-flight-or-fight actions, such as sexual reproduction, digestion, salivation, urination, and defecation.

Parkinson's disease is a degenerative disease of the central nervous system that causes shaking, rigidity, difficulty walking, and depression.

Pathogens are infectious agents such as viruses, bacteria, prions, fungi, viroids, or parasites.

Phagocytosis is the engulfing and digestion of cells, cellular material, and particles by other cells.

Phenotype is a composite of an organism's observable characteristics or traits.

Phosphorylation is the addition of a phosphate to an organic molecule. Phosphorylation generally activates proteins.

Picomole is a unit of substance in chemistry and physics that is equal to one trillionth (10^{-12}) of a mole.

piRNA or Piwi-RNA is the largest class of small noncoding RNA molecules expressed in animal cells. piRNA is involved in epigenetics and little is known about it.

Pituitary gland is a gland in the brainstem that releases a broad spectrum of hormones that control growth, blood pressure, thyroid function, metabolism, reproduction, osmotic homeostasis, kidney function, temperature regulation, and pain relief. Some of the hormones produced by the pituitary are human growth hormone (hGH), thyroid-stimulating hormone (TSH), adrenocorticotropic hormone (ACTH), β-endorphin prolactin (PRL), luteinizing hormone (LH), follicle-stimulating hormone (FSH), and melanocyte-stimulating hormone.

Placebo in medicine is a substance or procedure that causes an effect without having a specific activity for the condition being treated.

Plaques. Atherosclerotic plaques are found in blood vessels and are composed of accumulated white blood cells and lipids.

Plasmids are small DNA molecules that are physically separated from chromosomal DNA within a cell and can replicate independently. They are most commonly found in bacteria.

Polymerases (RNA and DNA) are enzymes that synthesize RNA during transcription and DNA polymerase synthesizes DNA during cellular replication.

Polymorphism is the occurrence of two or more different phenotypes in a given population.

Polypeptides are short chains of amino acids.

Positron emission tomography (PET) is a three-dimensional imaging technology based on introducing a positron-emitting radionuclide (tracer), which is introduced into the body attached to a biologically active molecule, and detecting the γ-radiation emitted.

Post-translational modification is a change in a protein that occurs after it is translated from RNA.

Post-traumatic stress syndrome (PTSD) is a condition that causes the reliving of traumatic events, avoidance of stressful events mimicking the trauma, and hyperarousal.

Prana is the Sanskrit word for vital energy or life force. Prana is the sum of all energy that is manifested in the universe.

Prefrontal cortex is the front part of the frontal lobe in the brain that is involved in complex cognition, personality, decision making, and social behavior.

Progesterone is a steroid involved in the menstrual cycle, pregnancy, and embryogenesis.

Promoter regions of genes are the regions near the transcription start site of a gene that allow for the binding of RNA polymerase in order to start transcription.

Prostasomes are membranous vesicles (40–500 nm in diameter) secreted by the prostate gland epithelial cells into seminal fluid.

Prostate cancer antigen 3 (PCA3) is a gene that expresses a noncoding RNA. PCA3 is only expressed in human prostate tissue, and the gene is highly overexpressed in prostate cancer. PCA3 RNA is useful as a tumor marker.

Prostate gland is a gland located between the bladder and penis of men. The prostate secretes fluid that nourishes and protects sperm.

Prostate-specific antigen (PSA) is a glycoprotein enzyme that is secreted by the prostate gland in men. PSA is present in small quantities in the serum of men with healthy prostates, but is often elevated in the presence of prostate cancer or other prostate disorders. Its purpose is to liquefy semen in order to allow sperm to swim freely.

Proteomics is the large-scale study of proteins, particularly their structures and functions.

Purines and pyrimidines are nitrogen-containing aromatic compounds that are found in DNA and RNA. The two-carbon nitrogen ring bases (adenine and guanine) are purines, while the one-carbon nitrogen ring bases (thymine, cytosine, and uracil) are pyrimidines.

Q

Qi is a traditional Chinese concept and is believed to be an active principle that forms part of any living thing. Qi literally translates as "breath," "air" and figuratively as "life force" or "energy flow."

Qigong is an ancient Chinese healthcare system that integrates physical postures, breathing techniques, and focused intention.

R

Randomized controlled trials (RCTs) are a type of scientific or medical experiment in which the people being studied are randomly assigned to one or another of the different treatments under study. The RCT is often considered the gold standard for a clinical trial.

Recessive genes are not expressed unless an individual received both copies of the recessive gene from each parent. An individual with one dominant and one recessive allele for a gene will have a dominant phenotype.

Recombinant DNAs are molecules formed by laboratory methods in order to bring together genetic material from multiple sources, creating sequences that are not found normally in biological organisms.

Recombination in genetics produces traits that differ from either parent. Genetic recombination occurs during meiosis and can lead to the creation of novel sets of genetic information that can be passed on to offspring.

Recommended daily allowance (RDA) is the daily dietary intake level of a nutrient that is considered sufficient by the Food and Nutrition Board of the Institute of Medicine.

It is revised every 5–10 years in order to make it easier for people to obtain their RDAs of each nutrient.

Regenerative or reparative medicine is a branch of research in tissue engineering and molecular biology that replaces, engineers, or regenerates human cells and tissues in order to restore normal function.

Reiki is a noninvasive human biofield therapy that was developed in 1922 by Japanese Buddhist Mikao Usui. It uses a technique commonly called hands-on-healing.

Replication. DNA replication is the process of producing two identical DNA molecules from one original DNA molecule and is the basis of the inheritance of our genes. DNA is made up of two strands, and each strand of the original DNA molecule serves as a template to create the complementary strand. DNA replication begins at origins of replication when the DNA unwinds, and DNA polymerases synthesize the two new DNAs by adding complementary nucleotides to the template strand.

Retinal pigment epithelium is the pigmented cell layer outside the neurosensory retina in the eye that nourishes retinal visual cells.

Retroviruses are single-stranded positive-sense RNA viruses with a DNA intermediate that target a host cell. Once inside the host cell, the virus uses its own reverse transcriptase enzyme in order to produce DNA from its RNA genome. This new DNA is then incorporated into the host cell genome by an integrase enzyme.

Rheumatoid arthritis is an autoimmune disease in which the immune system, which normally protects the body by attacking foreign substances such as bacteria and viruses, mistakenly attacks the joints.

Ribonucleic acid (RNA) is a polymeric molecule that is a nucleic acid that is essential for life. RNA has roles in the coding, decoding, regulation, and expression of genes.

RNA-induced silencing complex (RISC) is a multiprotein complex with a ribonucleoprotein that incorporates one strand of a double-stranded RNA fragment (such as siRNA or miRNA). The single strand acts as a template for the RISC to recognize the complementary mRNA transcript. The Argonaute proteins in the RISC activate and cleave the mRNA. This process is called RNA interference (RNAi) and is a key process in gene silencing.

RNA interference (RNAi) is an epigenetic process in which RNA inhibits gene expression, usually by causing the destruction of specific mRNAs.

RNA polymerase is an enzyme that produces the primary transcript RNA in transcription using DNA genes as a template.

Ribose is an organic compound with the formula $C_5H_{10}O_5$. It is formed from a pentose monosaccharide (a simple sugar).

Ribosomes are large and complex molecular machines in the cells that serve as the site for protein translation. Ribosomes link amino acids together in the order specified by the mRNA in order to create a polypeptide.

Rizatriptan is a drug for migraines.

RU486 is a steroid analog and potent antagonist of progesterone and glucocorticoids through its binding to their receptors.

S

Saccharin is an artificial sweetener with effectively no food energy.

Sanskrit is the primary liturgical language of Hinduism and a philosophical language in Buddhism, Hinduism, and Jainism.

Schizophrenia is a mental disorder characterized by abnormal social behavior along with a failure to recognize what is real. False beliefs, confused thinking, lack of motivation, auditory hallucinations, and reduced social interactions and emotional expression are common features of this disease.

Serotonin is a neurotransmitter. Biochemically derived from tryptophan, serotonin is primarily found in the gastrointestinal tract, blood platelets, and the central nervous system.

Single-nucleotide polymorphisms (SNPs) are variations in DNA sequences occurring commonly within a population in which a single nucleotide—A, T, C, or G—in the genome differs between members of a biological species or paired chromosomes.

Somatic nervous system is the part of the peripheral nervous system associated with skeletal muscle voluntary control of body movements.

Small interfering RNA (siRNA) is a class of double-stranded RNA that is involved in the RNA interference (RNAi) pathway, where it interferes with the expression of specific genes. siRNAs cause mRNA to be broken down after transcription and not translated into protein.

Spleen is an abdominal organ involved in the production and removal of blood and forms part of the immune system.

Splicing is a term in molecular biology and genetics in which there is a change in the pre-mRNA transcript so that introns are removed and exons are joined. This process occurs in the nucleus of the cell during transcription.

Stem cells are undifferentiated cells of a multicellular organism that give rise to more cells of one type, and from which other kinds of cells arise by differentiation.

> **Adult stem cells** are undifferentiated cells found throughout the body after development that divide in order to replenish dying cells and regenerate damaged tissues.

> **Embryonic stem cells (ESCs)** are pluripotent stem cells derived from the inner cell mass of a blastocyst, an early-stage preimplantation embryo. They have the ability to differentiate into any cell type and propagate.

> **Induced pluripotent stem cells (iPSCs)** are adult cells that have been genetically reprogrammed to an embryonic stem cell-like state by being forced to express genes and factors that are important for maintaining the properties of embryonic stem cells. They also have the ability to differentiate into any tissue. See Chapter 7 for the differences between ESCs and iPSCs.

Stroke is a physiological event in which poor blood flow to the brain results in cell death. There are two main types of stroke: ischemic due to a lack of blood flow, and hemorrhagic due to bleeding.

Stroma is part of a tissue that has a connective and structural role, but does not function as the main organ. It surrounds nerves, ducts, blood vessels, etc., and connects all of them in a tissue.

Sympathetic nervous system is one of the two main divisions of the autonomic nervous system (ANS). The other part of the ANS is the parasympathetic nervous system. The ANS functions to regulate the body's unconscious actions. The sympathetic nervous system's primary role is to stimulate the body's fight-or-flight response.

T

T lymphocytes are a type of lymphocyte, white blood cells that plays a central role in cell-mediated immunity.

Tachyarrhythmia is a resting heart rate that exceeds the normal resting rate. In general, a resting heart rate of over 100 beats per minute is accepted as tachyarrhythmia in adults.

Tai-Chi is a Chinese martial art practiced for both its defense training and its health benefits.

Tamoxifen is an antagonist of the estrogen receptor in breast tissue. Tamoxifen is the usual antiestrogen therapy for hormone receptor-positive breast cancer in premenopausal women, and is also a standard in postmenopausal women, although aromatase inhibitors are also frequently used.

Teratoma is a tumor with tissue or organ components resembling normal tissues derived from more than one germ layer.

Testicles are the male gonads in animals. Their primary functions are to produce sperm and to produce androgens, primarily testosterone.

Testosterone is a steroid hormone. In humans and other mammals, testosterone is secreted primarily by the testicles of males and, to a lesser extent, the ovaries of females. Small amounts are also secreted by the adrenal glands. It is the principal male sex hormone and an anabolic steroid.

Therapeutic Touch is a human biofield therapy or energy medicine technique that is based on ancient healing practices and was developed by Dr. Dorlores Kreiger and Dora Kunz in the 1970s.

Thymus is an organ that is part of the immune system and is where T cells (T lymphocytes) mature. T cells are part of the adaptive immune system, by which the body adapts specifically to foreign invaders.

Thyroid gland is a large gland that is found in the neck. The thyroid gland controls how quickly the body uses energy, makes proteins, controls the body's sensitivity to other hormones, and has a role in calcium homeostasis by producing and releasing specific hormones.

Tics are sudden, repetitive, non-rhythmic motor movements or vocalizations.

Titin, also known as connectin, is a very large protein that enables the elasticity of muscle.

Tonsils are masses of lymphatic material situated at either side of the back of the human throat.

Trans fats are a type of unsaturated fat that are uncommon in nature, but are also produced in the food industry from vegetable fats for use in margarine, snack food, packaged baked goods, and fried fast food.

Transcription is the mechanism by which genes are expressed. Transcription describes a process in which a particular segment of DNA is copied into mRNA.

Transgenes are genes or genetic materials that have been transferred naturally, or by genetic engineering techniques from one organism to another.

Transgenic mice contain additional, artificially introduced genetic material in every cell or a targeted group of cell types in a particular tissue. Transgenic mice are used to study specific genes of interest.

Translation is a part of gene expression in which the mRNA is decoded by a ribosome in order to produce a specific amino acid chain or polypeptide. This polypeptide will fold into an active protein in the cell and performs its function. The ribosome induces the binding of complementary transfer RNA (tRNA) anticodon sequences to mRNA codons. The tRNAs carry specific amino acids that are "read" by the ribosome, causing the amino acids to become chained together into a polypeptide.

Transposons are DNA sequences that changes their position in the genome.

Triglyceride is a blood lipid that transfers adipose fat and blood glucose from the liver in a bidirectional manner.

Triple-negative breast cancer is a type of breast cancer that does not express the genes for the estrogen receptor (ER), progesterone receptor (PR), or HER-2.

U

Ubiquitin is a small regulatory protein that has been found in almost all tissues. Ubiquitination is a post-translational modification in which ubiquitin is attached to a protein substrate. The addition of ubiquitin can affect proteins in many ways. It can signal for the protein's degradation via the proteasome, alter its cellular location, affect protein activity, and promote or prevent protein interactions.

Ultraviolet (UV) radiation is a form of electromagnetic radiation with a wavelength from 400 to 100 nm, which is shorter than that of visible light, but longer than that of x-rays.

V

Vasopressin, or antidiuretic hormone (ADH), is synthesized in the hypothalamus as a pre-prohormone precursor and stored in the pituitary, where it is released into the bloodstream. Vasopressin has two primary functions, which are to retain water in the body and to constrict blood vessels.

Ventricles are found in the heart and are two large chambers that collect and expel blood.

Vitamins (see Table 4.1 in Chapter 4) are organic compounds and vital nutrients that are required in limited amounts for proper functioning of the body.

W

World Health Organization (WHO) is a specialized agency of the United Nations (UN) that is concerned with international public health.

X

Xenotransplantation is a procedure that involves the transplantation, implantation, or infusion into a human of either: (a) live cells, tissues, or organs from a nonhuman animal source; or (b) human body fluids, cells, tissues, or organs that have had *ex vivo* contact with live nonhuman animal cells, tissues, or organs.

X-ray diffraction. DNA, unlike proteins, is an exceedingly large molecule that does not lend itself to crystallization, which is needed in the technique called x-ray crystallography. The structure of DNA was deduced by studying the x-ray diffraction patterns formed by DNA fibers kept at high humidity.

Y

Yamanka factors are Oct3/4, Sox2, Klf4, and c-Myc, which are highly expressed in embryonic stem cells (ESCs). Their overexpression can induce pluripotency in both mouse and human somatic cells, demonstrating that they can regulate the developmental signaling network necessary for creating ESCs.

Yoga is a physical, mental, and spiritual practice or discipline that originally came from India. Hatha yoga is a type of yoga with specific physical exercises (known as asanas or postures) and sequences of asanas, designed to align one's skin, muscles, and bones. The postures are also designed to open the many channels of the body, especially the spine, so that energy can flow freely in the body.

Index